The Only Way Out Is In

The Only Way Out Is In

Yoga, Ayurveda and Psychology

Reinhard Kowalski

JON CARPENTER

Our books may be ordered from bookshops or (post free) from
Jon Carpenter Publishing, Alder House, Market Street, Charlbury,
England OX7 3PH

Credit card orders should be phoned or faxed to 01689 870437
or 01608 811969

First published in 2001 by
Jon Carpenter
© Reinhard Kowalski 2001

Cover design by Reinhard Kowalski and Steve Jones

ISBN 1 897766 67 X

Printed in England by J. W. Arrowsmith Ltd., Bristol

Contents

Acknowledgements

Writing often feels like a very lonely activity. But it is not when I think of all the different parts of me that have been involved in the process, and all the different past and present experiences and energies that have flown through me into words. Then there are all the different people who have contributed, helped and challenged in the process of this book that started as an idea over three years ago. I should like to invite them all to join me here on this page to dedicate this book to you, the reader.

A special prayer of thanks is due to my teacher and Guru Paramahansa Yogananda, whose work has inspired me to write these pages. I am also grateful to Self-Realization Fellowship in Los Angeles for permission to use quotes from the work of Paramahansa Yogananda and from other SRF publications. Thanks to Sister Nivedita of SRF for taking the time to read and meet with me and discuss at the SRF Convocation 2000 in Los Angeles. I also want to acknowledge the energy of all the 4000 people at the SRF Convocation in 1997 where the idea for this book was born. Thanks to Maryann Miller who was the first person who listened to the idea on that occasion.

Thank you to my friends Nick and Helena Lovendal-Duffell for their continuous encouragement and for sharing their wonderful place in France, where these last words are written. Thanks to the Swamis and monks at the Vedanta Centre in Bourne End for having me on 'writing retreats', and thanks to all the members of the London SRF group for having provided a spiritual home. Thanks to Karl and Ursula Furrer of the Swiss Health Resort in California for providing the peace for the last chapter.

I thank especially Jane Ingram for reading, correcting and querying the whole manuscript. And thanks to Penny Tyndale-Hardy, Corinna Jurk and especially Veronica Houghton for reading, commenting and encouragement.

Thanks to all of you who have helped me turn these thoughts into a practical service for others as MindBalancing meditation groups for staff in the Health Service, especially Corinne Usher, Jacob John, Gill Wilkie, Clive Stevenson, Linda Lloyd, Veronica Lovelace, Jeanie Reeve, Peter Harding and all my colleagues and friends in the South Buckinghamshire NHS Trust. Also thanks to the members of my meditation group who have listened to the draft versions of MindBalancing. Special thanks to those who are assisting me in running the groups, in particular Elizabeth Smith, Bhavna Jani-Negandhi, Lyn Lidiard and

Brenda Deller. Thanks to Steve Jones for his creativity and patience in recording the audio-tape and helping with the cover design.

Ayurveda is an key ingredient of the book. Special thanks to David Frawley for inspiring me and writing the foreword. Thanks also to Vasant Lad and his Ayurvedic Institute for stimulating my interest in Ayurveda and psychology.

Thanks to Jon Carpenter, my publisher, for taking on me and this book.

Thank you all and bless you all!

Reinhard Kowalski, Jouqueviel, February 2001

Foreword

Psychology could be called the religion of the modern world, at least for the developed world and its intellectual elite. We are all analyzing ourselves, our behavior and our relationships, whether at home, at work, or in our travels. Psychology is our way of looking at our psyche and trying to initiate changes in our consciousness so that we can become happier and more complete. The psychologist is often like a priest who provides a prescription for self-improvement, peace and forgiveness. Counseling is a way of communing with the hidden side of our nature and exorcising negative behavioral patterns that waylay us from the dark.

Psychology offers us a way to objectively examine our consciousness. It shows us how to work on ourselves. It is not limited to faith or ritual. It does not give us a savior to solve our problems or to redeem our sins by proxy. It places the problem and its solution in our own hands.

In fact, one could argue that psychology today is part of a new spirituality that is trying to emerge, a way of self-realisation, as opposed to the old way of subordination to an external deity or church. The religions of the world have also begun to reformulate themselves in a modern psychological language, which affords them a much greater appeal and usefulness. Naturally, as psychology grows it will expand to integrate more spiritual tools into its practice. This has taken Western psychology in the direction of Eastern spirituality. Yet the encounter with Eastern spirituality also involves seeing the limitations of Western psychology, which after all is a new discipline that is scarcely a century old. It also involves a cultural critique, seeing how the psychological state of our culture, which can be neurotic, influences, creates or upholds our personal disturbances.

Eastern – or what we could call yogic spirituality – is also a psychology, but this is only its first step. It examines our personal psychology in order to take us beyond it to the personal and the cosmic. It shows us how to transcend our human psychology into a higher consciousness through which we can observe or witness our psychology and no longer be ruled by it. This does not mean that our particular psychological patterns go away entirely, any-more than the shape of our bone structure changes, but that we learn how to use our psychology in a positive manner. It is like a scorpion whose stinger has been removed.

Integrating psychology East and West is an important and complex topic that brings us face to face with the most profound questions of life. The Eastern world has a much deeper and more spiritual idea of the psyche. It brings past lives, higher states of consciousness and occult powers into the arena of the mind. It offers powerful tools of yoga and meditation to change the mind, including working with the breath and the senses. Yet with all of this the East is often psychologically naïve on a personal level and has little sense of the role of emotions in mental health. It can ignore or suppress the human dimension for family, social or religious ties, in which the individual gets suppressed and is unable to transcend.

For traditional Orientals, like Hindus and Buddhists, devotion to a guru or a deity is the panacea for all psychological problems from fear to grief, from anxiety to depression. Such a prescription may work but is hard for Western people, trained in science, to accept. Clearly an adaptation is required. We must recognize our personal dimension and give it its place. On the other hand, we must not let it dominate us or become the be all of our culture. We must adapt yogic tools in a way that is meaningful for us on a personal and cultural level.

Many people in the West who begin to follow Eastern meditation paths get stuck in their own unresolved emotions and subconscious patterns arising from childhood, which they project upon the guru or the path, just as they may project these upon the therapist. The meditation generation has also been the baby boomers, the broken family generation, and the self-assertion generation. That is not the best foundation for spiritual practice that requires selflessness and peace.

Reinhard Kowalski is a psychotherapist by training who has a solid footing of many years on the yogic path. He is a devotee of Paramahansa Yogananda, perhaps the greatest yogi to come to the West, whose teachings offer an integral path of meditation, pranayama, devotion and service that provides a balanced and wholesome development for anyone who takes it up with sincerity. Kowalski reflects Yogananda's balanced approach and adds a psychological dimension to make it more relevant to people today.

As the book's wonderful title so amply proclaims, 'the only way out is in'. There is no real outer solution to our personal problems. There is no ultimate joy in accumulating the things of the world, like wealth or position, however helpful these may be in making our outer life easier. In fact, they can be a trap, an outer allure or complication that prevents us from looking within. All our trials and tribulations that are a cause of so much upset and agitation are really heavenly messengers telling us that the outer world is not the true reality, that our outer being is not our true Self. The only way out in any lasting sense is to dive deep within our own minds and heart.

Reinhard Kowalski provides an excellent bridge between the best in Western psychology and the most relevant in yogic spirituality. He has worked with practical tools in both fields and shows how to blend them in a harmonious manner. He points out the relevance of meditation, pranayama, mantra and devotion as psychological tools, showing how to use them to change our thoughts, emotions and deep-seated conditionings. His book is a practical guide on how yogic tools can be employed for psychological transformation, so that we can once and for all be free from all our intractable negative emotional patterns and reclaim our immortal joy and creativity in life.

Such an East-West translation is not easy. It is not an academic task but one that must be done in one's own daily life. The book reflects the profound inner journey of the author and how he has learned to transform himself. It also shows how he has been able to transform his profession into spiritual work, affording a much deeper level of help to his clients. Reinhard Kowalski uses his own personal spiritual journey as a metaphor for psychological and spiritual change and shows how other people can follow a similar path.

This book is all about how to turn psychological difficulties into spiritual opportunities. It also shows how to overcome the psychological difficulties that all travelers on the spiritual path must confront at one time or another, their dark night of the soul. It is both for those seeking psychological healing and for those seeking spiritual growth.

The Only Way Out Is In should be read by all psychologists, meditators and yoga teachers to help them understand how to use their practices for an integral transformation of body, mind and spirit. It is a breakthrough work in East-West psychological studies that moves from the realm of theory into that of practical application. Most importantly, it provides a wealth of simple methods that any person can use on a daily basis to fundamentally improve the quality of their consciousness.

Dr. David Frawley (Pandit Vamadeva Shastri)
Author, *Yoga and Ayurveda, Ayurveda and the Mind*, and *Vedantic Meditation*
Ayurvedic doctor, Vedic astrologer, Vedic teacher
Director of the American Institute of Vedic Studies in Santa Fe, New Mexico.

We Want to Get Out

We want to get out
out of this ageing body,
out from behind the prison bars
of aching bones.

We feel separated
inside this body,
held in by skin, bones and flesh,
lonely inside our cell.

Our thoughts and feelings
circle around in the dark chamber
of our psyche,
often overpowering,
often making us feel so lonely.

So we drink the outside in through our senses,
meeting others through words, touch and sex,
eating, smoking, drinking,
all attempts to bring the outside in – somehow.
Words, thoughts, sex to merge with someone – somehow.

We want to merge,
so desperately,
but we don't know how.
The longing is so great,
the attempts are so futile.

And all this – an illusion?
And all this – a dream?
The illusion of maya,
the loneliness we have created ourselves.
In reality we are all one,
in reality we are all connected,
the wise ones say.

Our thoughts and feelings

can fly freely through time and space,
dancing with others in this universe.
The temporary shell of our body,
grown from the same matter
that makes the earth and the galaxies,
is just another thought in the mind of creation.

We are all one,
but aware mainly of our separateness.
Deep, deep inside us there is this place
where we can feel and be this one-ness.
Deep, deep inside us our soul is waiting
to lead us on our blissful dance through the universe.

Introduction

With this book I am trying to introduce a new psychology, which is based in Ayurveda and yoga. The book is both theoretical and practical. As David Frawley suggests in his foreword, you can use it as a workbook for your own psycho-spiritual development. Or you can use it to explore new ways of thinking about psychology.

The book contrasts and explores two fundamentally different ways of being. These two polarised ways form the basis for this new psychology. The two modes of being are:

1 The focus of one's life on sense-gratification, and all the personality characteristics that this entails.
2 A way of being that sees life-energy as essentially God-given, and that must therefore be used in a balanced way rather than just being pushed into the senses.

At a practical level this book is about the way inside to soul. It is written for people who want to get out of the superficiality of their everyday lives, out of many of the senseless stresses and strains of work and home, out of habitual attachments and addictions, and ultimately out of malaise and depression. Our world is full of superficiality, stress, addictions and depression. Our world even seems to depend on it. The only way out is in. But we need maps for the journey to soul. We need to understand ourselves, the world we live in, and the way our mind works, because we need the mind's co-operation (understanding) for the journey. The models that you will find on the following pages are therefore psychological and spiritual mind maps to help you gain a different understanding and thus free your blocked intuition. The treasure soul is hidden, not in the external achievements of the ego, but in the chambers of silence and stillness within. The models that follow will hopefully help you on your journey to your own inner sanctuary, which is the place from which you can approach the outside world in a soul-directed way.

This book tries to speak directly to you, even when it does not address you directly. It tries to speak to your mind, your heart and your soul. It tries to convince your intellectual mind that going inside is not only a good idea, but also essential for your future well-being. It pleads with your intellectual mind to make some space for the intuitive mind which is the voice of the soul. Your intellect is important in this process. In my model it is the intellect that can pave the way for the journey away from external superficialities to internal depth. Once you begin to 'feel' that the only way out is in, then you know that your soul's intuition is beginning to express itself.

This journey is not easy, because it asks you to question many ideas that you have about yourself and the world around you. It asks you to trust something that, so far, you might not even know exists. To begin with, therefore, I have to ask you to trust me.

When people come to see me for psychotherapy they usually do not know me. They may have heard something about me from somebody; or they may trust somebody's recommendation. Usually they then trust me when they come to see me. That trust is absolutely essential for therapy to work. I feel honoured by that trust, and I hope that I can be worthy of it.

But all you have is a book – words written on paper by someone you probably do not know. You may have been attracted by the title. Whatever your motives are, I should like you to know that my motivation for writing this book has come out of my work with myself and with my clients. The book wants to be of service and it includes my prayers and meditations, which will hopefully reach you as healing energy on your path.

The material for this book has accumulated over the past few years and it has grown out of my own journey and out of my work with my clients. It is the book that I would like to give to all my clients. It is meant to help you go behind, beyond and underneath your struggles and your suffering so that you can find your way to that inner wealth you have, which is called soul.

Please feel free to skip certain chapters if you find them too theoretical. Especially Chapters 5 and 6 may feel like that, because they explore some Western psychological models in some detail. However, please do try to digest Chapter 7, because it contains the central model for most of my considerations.

1
Psychology, Cosmology and Religion

This book is about religion and psychology. This is not as strange a combination as it may seem, if you consider that both disciplines are concerned with finding meaning in life, death, suffering, pain. Basically they are about finding a deeper (or higher) meaning above or below our direct experience of existence. The religious or spiritual models I shall be using are based in yoga and Ayurveda, which are both part of the ancient Indian philosophical and healing sciences. Yoga here is meant in its proper meaning as the spiritual and psychological science that originates in the ancient Indian Vedas. Yoga is the path to achieve union with God.

Please do not let your confused feelings or even repulsion against the word 'religion' turn you off from reading on. It will all make sense in the end, just as it has all made sense to me over the years. In one short book I am trying to present to you what has taken me many years of work as a psychotherapist to figure out. My own and others' searching and suffering form the context for this book. My intention is to help you along with your searching and through your suffering.

Religion has received a somewhat 'bad name' in our rational, scientific world of production and consumption. We have become caught in the illusion that our scientists have got it all pretty much sussed. We believe that the way we see the world is how it is. That it's all pretty much sorted and that it is just a question of time before science will have solved the few remaining mysteries. But science, all over the place, is discovering more mysteries and paradoxes that make many of our dearly held beliefs questionable.

Einstein and his theories are often used by the 'new science movement' and by cosmologists (like, for example, Brian Swimme) to explain how the official view of 'the universe and everything' is changing. This very much includes our (yours and mine) place in our universe.

Let us take an example. Originally it was thought that the Earth was the centre of the universe with all the stars circling around us. Copernicus then discovered that we were not the centre at all. The Earth moves around the Sun with a bunch of other planets. Our solar system is part of our Milky Way galaxy which has billions of stars like our sun. Our galaxy is part of the Virgo super-cluster of galaxies, and there are billions of galaxies with billions of stars each. The distances between stars and galaxies are millions and billions of light-years. We are just one tiny spot in the vastness of the universe. That realisation certainly put us in our place.

But now the view is changing again. Cosmologists have discovered that it is all far more complicated. Time and space ('space-time') are more mysterious and complex than previously thought. The agreement now seems to be that we and everything else in the universe are all at the centre of it. Our universe has a 'multiplicity of centres'. Ultimately each one of us, each cell and atom and particle, is right there at the centre of it all.

> Every place in the universe is at the center of this exploding reality. From our place on Earth today in the midst of the Virgo Supercluster, all of the universe explodes away from us, just as it does from the perspective of anyone in the Perseus Supercluster. We are at the unmoving center of this cosmic expansion, and we have been here at the center from the beginning of time.[1]

So it is not too far out to assume that we all might have a centre of the universe right here inside ourselves. It boggles the mind because it throws our usual way of thinking about space and time into confusion. 'Stay with the confusion and the mystery of it all', cosmologists like Brian Swimme say, 'because through the mystery the story of the universe is revealing itself'. And we are part of that mystery. Our whole being, even our thoughts, cannot be separated from the stars, the galaxies and all the processes that go on in our universe. But to see it like that, to feel, to experience it like that, many of our well-established patterns of seeing and thinking need to be changed. We have even grown out of the habit of seeing ourselves as part of planet Earth. We have turned our planet and her other creatures into sub-human 'things' to be exploited and dominated by us. So we need to start by seeing ourselves again as an integral part of our planet, before we can venture into experiencing ourselves as part of the cosmos. The message is that we need to widen our perspective and our horizon.

Another example would be the model of 'quantum vacuum'. Basically it says that space or vacuum is far from empty. It is full of elementary particles that suddenly appear from nowhere.

> These elementary particles crop up out of the vacuum itself – that is the simple and awesome discovery. I am asking you to contemplate a universe where, somehow, being itself arises out of a field of 'fecund emptiness'.[2]

All this gets very religious in a way. There seems to be something beyond matter, something mysterious, intangible, energy that seems to be creating everything including time and space and even us. And we are right in the middle of it. Material things are not as solid as they seem to be, and there is something happening within us, between us and between us and everything else that has to do with emptiness and light and energy. Ultimately it stresses the power of subtle energies like light, sound and even thought in the process of creation.

God

Does this then mean that we have to believe in God, in a creator? No, we don't have to, because we have free will. However, it seems that recent scientific disciplines like nuclear physics, quantum physics and cosmology, often called 'the new science movement', are all pointing towards the existence of a higher creative power beyond the world of matter. It seems that the split between religion and science that we have grown used to is disappearing. In my psychotherapy practice I find that increasing numbers of people are disillusioned with the 'progress' that humanity has created on our planet and are asking rather spiritual questions about the meaning of their lives.

Religion is about the seeking of bliss or happiness – all the religions of the world do not differ much in this. Psychotherapy is also about finding happiness. Both religion and psychotherapy therefore have theories about the origins of pain and suffering.

There is an ancient, some say the oldest, religion on this planet that has a philosophy and a view of the universe and creation that matches all the latest findings and assumptions from cosmology and from quantum physics. Its sacred scriptures, the Vedas, were originally passed on orally in verse for thousands of years and are said to predate recorded history. This religion has a clear philosophical and psychological framework to explain the origins of pain and suffering; and it gives clear practical steps for achieving bliss and happiness. It even has a complex and holistic system of physical and psychological healing methods called Ayurveda. The religion is Hinduism, and the ancient Vedas, assumed to date back to 6,000 BC, are the holy scriptures that in parts speak almost the same language as the 'new' scientists do. Hinduism has a very definite concept of God and a rather practical approach to him. It says that every human being's aim in life is to uncover his soul so that the soul can go about its business of re-connecting with God. The very practical science for this is yoga.

> Hinduism is a vast and profound religion. It worships one Supreme Reality (called by many names) and teaches that all souls ultimately realize Truth. There is no eternal hell, no damnation. It accepts all genuine spiritual paths … . Each soul is free to find his own way, whether by devotion, austerity, meditation (yoga) or selfless service. … Hinduism is a mystical religion, leading the devotee to personally experience the Truth within, finally reaching the pinnacle of consciousness where man and God are one.[3]

At this point I should like to give you an example for the rather comprehensive theory of creation that can be found in the Vedas. Paramahansa Yogananda says the following about the three aspects of nature in an article that was written in 1934 about how the early rishis (seers) of India went about trying to find God.

> Worship of God in prehistoric times began through man's fear of the various forces of nature. When it rained excessively, floods killed many people. Awed, man thought of rain and wind and other natural forces as gods.
>
> Later on, human beings realized that nature operates in three ways: creative, preservative, and dissolutive. A wave rising out of the ocean exemplifies the creative state; staying for a moment on the sea-breast, it is in the preservative state; and sinking back into the deep, it passes through the dissolutive state.
>
> Just as Jesus beheld the universal forces of evil personified in Satan, so the great rishis beheld the universal forces of creation, preservation, and dissolution personified in definite forms. The sages of old named them Brahma the Creator, Vishnu the Preserver, and Shiva the Destroyer. These primal powers were created as projections of the unmanifested Spirit to unfold His infinite drama of creation, while He, as God beyond creation, remains ever hidden behind their consciousness. In times of cosmic dissolution, all creation and its vast activating forces dissolve back into Spirit. There they rest until called upon again by the Great Director to re-enact their roles.[4]

I should like to make it clear where I am coming from. Initially this book started off with what is now Chapter 2, and I tried to gradually phase in terms like soul and spirit. The word God I tried to avoid altogether, because it felt embarrassing and because I did not want to turn those readers off who do not believe in God. So I tried to sneak it in through the back door. At some point I had to question my motives for this. Why does it feel odd to write openly about God? Is it because the God we know is the one that the Christian church presents us with at our occasional visits? Not very popular, not very trendy, is it? Even when they try to dress it all up with pop and rock music, it still feels stale and stuffy, very abstract and not practical at all. Or is it because God really doesn't fit into our ever so rational and scientific approach to the world? Or is it all because of my own ambivalence? It certainly has not been easy for me to come to terms with a concept of devotion to God, even though I remember feeling very devoted to God as a child.

My relationship with God or the concept of God has been an on-and-off affair, as for so many of us. I remember I was talking to him when I was 10. Prayer was then part of the way in which I was trying to deal with the loneliness of an only child, and with many issues that required guidance that was not forthcoming from my parents. I felt bad when I missed a Sunday at my Lutheran church in Germany. By the time Confirmation happened at 14, God had faded somewhat into the background – adolescence and girls were taking up most of my mental and physical space. However, there still was a relationship there. Then, a few years later, I was privileged to go for one year as an exchange student to the USA. My year was organised through International Christian Youth Exchange and I was sponsored by the First Congregational Church in a small town in Massachusetts. Regular Sunday church services and participation in all sorts of church events were part of my year. I even wrote a prayer which I read out at a Christmas service. I used newspaper headlines, which at the time were mainly about the war in Vietnam. I should like to share this prayer with you.

Let us pray.
Father,
We are standing before you. Some of us are tired, some of us are bored.
We are your congregation.
We are standing before you with all our common and personal problems.
We cannot judge most of these problems. But do not let this disability be an excuse for being unconcerned.
'L.B.J. sends Congress war-swollen budget.'
'Deadly Soviet mine makes Viet debut.'
Father, remind us that we must help.
Remind us that you showed us the way and that we have to walk by ourselves.

'North Korea Ambush killed 6 U.S. soldiers.'
'War to bitter end, pledged by Hanoi.'
Father, in spite of this news, let us not continue to be peacemakers by fooling ourselves with the notion that it is always 'the bad guys against the good guys.'

'Hanoi insisted – stop bombing.'
'U.S. hints, Viet Cong could attend parley.'
Remind us that you created all mankind in your own image.

'Body of Framingham boy found in Sudbury River.'
'Springfield gets a black eye in race discrimination study.'
Father, remind us that Jesus is given to all of us and that we cannot keep him carefully hidden behind our Sunday church necktie.
Let us realise that the other guy knows about him too.

Remind us that this prayer is going to be one of those innocent, empty sayings, if we do not realise that Vietnam, poverty, and racial discrimination surround everyone of us and that everyone of us is exactly the right one to do something about it.
Father, let us not overestimate this quoting, Bible-repeating, long-playing record, on

which many of us have written the words Jesus and Christianity. Let us realise that
Jesus primarily is in our lives and that secondarily we worship him in his church.
Remind us that we have to decide now what we can do.
Let us not get used to our sweet indifferent selves.

Amen.

The political connection in the prayer is clearly there. Vietnam and Simon and Garfunkel were stirring our adolescent hearts. After my return to Germany, many of my American schoolfriends went to fight in that senseless war. One of them came back only to drown himself in Boston harbour. What horrors he must have seen. At high school he had been one of the softest, most intelligent and most sensitive boys in my class. I can still see his big brown eyes under dark bushy eyebrows and his slightly absent soft smile.

The prayer is full of devotion, crying out for social justice and urging people and me to do something about injustice. I now ask myself what happened to all that devotion? Why was there nobody who could channel it in the right direction? The prayer also shows the limitations of my understanding of God at the time: *Let us realise that Jesus primarily is in our lives and that secondarily we worship him in his church.* To have Jesus in one's life meant doing good, fighting against war and injustice. For me, and for most other Christians to this day, it has little to do with a practical scientific method of getting to know God, having a personal relationship with him. And the church had not much to say about fighting injustice either. So we were really left with worshipping in church once a week.

The Christian church I knew had very little to say about the state of the world, about wars and politics, and I never understood why. Back in Germany I made friends with people who were involved in Marxist groups. Teachers introduced me to philosophy and literature, a lot of it Marxist and socialist and dealing with Germany's turbulent and cruel recent past. Suddenly I was beginning to find models that helped me understand my father's struggles. After all, he was a coal-miner, a member of the oppressed working class. Marxism helped me understand his unhappiness. God became a dubious figure who, listening to his representatives in the Christian churches, had not much to say about the things that were important to me. There was no view of the world, no relevant philosophy, no goal. Marxism made more sense of my life. Then at university in West Berlin I began to feel that the world could be changed. That world that had caused so much misery for my father and people like him. Something needed to be done, and Marxism and the socialist state next door (East Germany) showed what could be done. There was hope. The God of the Christian Church never offered that kind of clarity and action plan. God and church were always somewhat removed from reality, and therefore easy to forget in the struggles and the excitements of everyday. Religion was reserved for Sundays, Easter and Christmas, but even then other things became more real, more important.

I now know that I faced one of the big shortcomings of our culture. Reality was scientific, rational, practical, and even exciting and romantic. Religion was for certain rituals, birth, marriage and death, and mainly for old people, because they were on the way out, while I was on the way in. Within myself I was feeling the split between the secular and the celestial that is in reality fairly new in human history and that has taken off only with industrialisation.

Many people are now beginning to voice that feeling of the un-naturalness of this split and are trying to remedy it. Science, rationality and practicality are not delivering the bliss they promised. Disillusionment is widespread, but at the same time we seem to keep God locked up behind the doors of churches and underneath piles of high-tech Christmas presents.

An article in the *Sunday Times* (14.12.1997) says a lot about the Christian church's dilemma. The headline reads *Pope builds telescope to find God*. Apparently the Vatican is sponsoring a telescope to try and find the 'fingerprints of God amid the chaos of the cosmos. ... For the Vatican, maintaining a team of astronomers is seen as vital to prevent repeats of its past battles with scientists. ... Father Chris Corbally, an English Jesuit who is the observatory's deputy director, said: 'If civilisations were to be found on other planets and if it were feasible to communicate, then we would want to send missionaries to save them, just as we did in the past when new lands were discovered.''

I have to say I find this story, if correctly reported, very worrying because it is so ignorant, contradictory and simplistic. Modern science is discovering patterns and mysteries. It is not about finding fingerprints amid chaos, but about connecting with the power behind and within the patterns and mysteries. It is also not about preventing repeats of past battles between church and science, but about acknowledging and exploring the church's dogmatic ignorance and science's dogmatic arrogance that led to the battles. And then – we are going to save aliens. Just as we, in the past, 'saved' Native Americans, Australian Aborigines, Mayas, Incas, and countless other people who were quite happy with their mostly extremely wise and practical religions? I find this statement very frightening.

Finding a Guru – Paramahansa Yogananda

A book like this one is always subjective as well as objective. Actually, this is another revelation from nuclear physics, where it was found that the subjective and the objective cannot really be separated. In nuclear physics this applies to the relationship between the observer and the movement of particles. I think the same is true in my field of psychotherapy, where the suffering that each individual brings to me cannot be separated from my own suffering and from the suffering of humanity as a whole. Jung used the term 'collective unconscious' to refer to our inter-connectedness at the subconscious level. I would go even further and claim that individuality and separation are an illusion and that we are all floating in one collective soup with everything we do, feel, and think. Consequently my story and many of my clients' stories over twenty years are part of this book, even in the parts that seem to be objective.

The basic premise of this book and the path that it wants to lead to, are based in the teachings of Paramahansa Yogananda, whom I should like to introduce to you at this stage.

After taking my psychology degree in West Berlin I came to England and trained in Behaviour Therapy and in Clinical Psychology. During my career as a clinical psychologist in the National Health Service I reached a state of burn-out and as a result trained in psychosynthesis psychotherapy in the mid 1980s. Psychosynthesis, which will be referred to repeatedly later, became my first intro-duction to psycho-spiritual approaches to therapy. There followed many years of spiritual searching and a great deal of confusion. Teachers, supervisors and ther-apists became pseudo-gurus, and many of them seemed to quite enjoy their role. While my clients were projecting wisdom and all-knowing perfection onto me, thus flattering my ego, I was doing the same with my teachers and therapists. My spiritual path got lost in the jungle of therapy dressed up as spirituality. In the process I learnt a lot about myself and became, I think and hope, quite a good psychotherapist. But something was still missing. Often I carried all the drama and despair that my clients brought to me. Often I went into deep states of anxiety and depression. The answer was always – more work on myself, just resolving this additional bit of childhood trauma, more therapy, more training courses, more intense digging around in the dark depths of the subconscious.

Then, one day, I felt in a deep crisis yet again (or was it the same crisis just slowly deepening?), when a book fell off the shelf in a bookshop right in front of my feet. It was Paramahansa Yogananda's *The Divine Romance*. I bought the book and started reading. I loved the style and it felt like the words were speaking directly to me. It all was beginning to fall into place. I got quite excited about many of the chapter titles: A new look at the origin and nature of cosmic creation; Practising religion scientifically; Psychological furniture; How feelings mask the soul; Ridding the consciousness of worry. There were many of the answers, and connections between psyche and spirit, that I had been looking for. I started to systematically study Yogananda's teachings and I began to practise his very structured meditation, concentration and yoga exercises. Slowly but steadily I found myself on a spiritual path and in my therapy work I was beginning to include more and more spiritual elements. This book is a result of the process.

Paramahansa Yogananda was born in India in 1893 and died in Los Angeles in 1952. After graduating from Calcutta University in 1915 he became a monk of India's Swami Order. He founded a spiritually orientated school in India and went to the United States in 1920 to speak at a congress of religious leaders on the topic 'the science of religion'. That same year he founded Self-Realization Fellowship as an international society to disseminate his teachings on the science, philosophy and practice of yoga and meditation, and to integrate the spiritual traditions of East and West. Yogananda's organisation has continued to grow even after his death and is continuing to publish and practise his teachings, which are based in Eastern philosophy, in a way that is easily digestible for Westerners (see SRF address in 'Advice and Resources' for further information).

The writings of Paramahansa Yogananda show that science and religion do not have to be in conflict. He also shows that essentially all religions are the same, and that it is a very practical matter.

> The essential point to be remarked about Paramahansa Yogananda's teaching, in contradistinction to that of European philosophers such as Bergson, Hegel, and others, is that it is not speculative, but practical, even when dealing with the utmost reaches of metaphysics. The reason is that the Hindus, alone of mankind, have penetrated behind the veil, and possess the knowledge, which is really not philosophical, i.e. wisdom-loving, but wisdom itself.[5]

Personally I have found in Yogananda's teachings a very practical spiritual path which includes devotion to God as an important element. Because of my strong initial scepticism I am only now beginning to understand why devotion is important, and I shall share my understanding of it later in this book. The spiritual path advocated by Yogananda is based in the Hindu Vedic tradition and includes a range of meditation and yoga techniques, which all aim at going inside to the soul and thus have a direct experience of spirit, God and cosmic bliss. The techniques are all based in a sound framework of metaphysical theory.

I have now been practising the techniques and studying the teachings for some years, and this has, of course, influenced my work as a psychotherapist. My doubts about certain psychotherapy models and practices have grown and my own practice has changed, with very positive results for me and my clients. I have become convinced that the only way out is in.

2

Yoga and Ayurveda

How can we make sense of it? Something seems to be wrong – with ourselves, our relationships, society, politics, values. Everything is becoming faster, everybody wants more, all the time. Wasn't technology meant to make life easier for everybody? Wasn't science meant to create food and well-being for all? We suffer the questions and don't believe in answers any longer. Brother Achalananda, a minister of Self-Realization Fellowship, asks similar questions:

> Why are most people today in such a rush that they cannot even find time to relax and cultivate relationships with their spouse and children, much less with God? Economic reasons and the sheer complexity of modern life explain to a certain extent why people are so frantic, but beyond these there is something deeper: the fact that their lifestyles leave certain basic needs unfulfilled. By crowding their daily schedules with more work, more entertainment, more of all kinds of outer activity, people are desperately trying to find a way to fill the tremendous sense of emptiness they feel within.[6]

This implies that there is a connection between our increasingly frantic life and our inner emptiness. It seems to make sense: we are searching for something, can't find it, so we search more, all the while not realising that we are searching in the wrong place. But why would we not realise that we are searching in the wrong place? The human intellect has made the most amazing discoveries. Why then would such a relatively simple question not attract the attention of our intellectual powers? Why are there not millions of people on this planet shouting: *Stop, we are looking in the wrong place*? Why is it so difficult not to get caught in the frantic cycle of wanting, buying, consuming, wanting more?

Marxism would see it all as an inevitability in the development of capitalism. But, as we shall see later, that is only part of the story. There is a more universal process underneath. The Hindu model of the Yugas, very long life cycles of our planet, offers a fascinating explanation. It says that our whole planet moves through four different stages of development, each lasting between 1,200 and 4,800 years, in ascending and descending cycles (see Sri Yukteswar, *The Holy Science*, for more details). According to this cosmology we have just (at around

1700 A.D.) moved out of Kali Yuga (the iron or dark ages) into Dwapara Yuga (the bronze or atomic age) in an ascending cycle leading, in thousands of years, to a new Satya Yuga (golden age).

> ...We really have left behind the period of grossest materialism, Kali Yuga, and are quite far into the beginnings of Dwapara Yuga, the next stage in the ascending cycle. As we move into this atomic age, more and more of the finer forces of nature that were unknown in the Dark Ages are beginning to be harnessed, giving rise to global telecommunications, computers, advances in medicine, agriculture, transportation – all those technologies that are so radically changing the fabric of daily life. However, the Kali Yuga from which we have just emerged is still a very strong influence. Because of this, our culture tends still to use scientific advances not only to do good, but also to cater to our grosser materialistic instincts of selfishness, destruction, greed.[7]

The model of the Yugas can certainly explain the global contradictions and our inability to see clearly, both of which we experience so acutely. This book goes a step further and tries to explore the psychological dynamics of this global situation, while also trying to guide your mind step by step towards a new understanding of yourself and the universe. It wants to be psychological, philosophical and practical.

Unfortunately most Western psychological models have not much to offer when it comes to explaining the dynamics of the outside world, let alone the universe as a whole. Equally unfortunately the new models in cosmology and quantum physics that were referred to in the introduction usually lack psychological depth. The ancient yogic writings of the East, on the other hand, give us models and theories that explain creation as a complex process of differentiation from the very beginning down to our present inner and outer worlds, identifying the same patterns at each different level. You may want to ask how the rishis, the originators of these ancient texts, knew all this thousands of years ago. Apparently they lived in a previous 'golden age', when such knowledge was easily available through yogic practices. I do not want to argue the validity of this assumption here, but rather show throughout the book how this ancient knowledge does seem to pull together and expand many of the disconnected strands of Western psychology and cosmology.

Therefore, in order to be psychological, philosophical and practical we need to build a bridge between Western psychological thinking and yogic holistic thinking. I shall in particular focus on Ayurveda, the 'science of life', which is the healing branch of the ancient Indian Vedic wisdom and closely connected with the spiritual science of yoga. I strongly believe that since we are living in times of such enormous inner and outer paradoxes and challenges, such a bridge between East and West is becoming vital for our psychological and spiritual healing.

Western psychology has amassed enormous knowledge about ego-development and about the subconscious. But we have now reached a stage in our evolution where we are challenged to go beyond the subconscious into the superconscious; beyond the healing of past trauma towards our spiritual destiny; beyond what psychotherapy has to offer, on to the experience of ourselves as little soul-waves that want to re-unite with the ocean of spirit. Western psychotherapy does not go beyond the ego and the sense-mind; it tries to help people achieve bliss and happiness within the world of duality. According to Vedic wisdom this state of bliss is not possible without re-connecting with the soul first.

Ayurveda and Sankhya

At this point I should like to introduce the basic concepts of Ayurvedic cosmology that form the implicit basis for this book. Ayurveda is based in the Sankhya system, which is one of the classical schools of Vedic philosophy. This is closely connected with Patanjali's *Yoga Sutras* and also with the *Bhagavad Gita*. A lot of my writing in this book has been inspired by Paramahansa Yogananda's commentary on the *Bhagavad Gita*.[8] However, I am approaching the Ayurvedic and yogic concepts from a Western psychological perspective. This means that the Ayurvedic concepts of the mind and the ego are implicitly present throughout the following chapters, but mostly not explicitly referred to. David Frawley presents in his books a very detailed Ayurvedic analysis of the mind (see Notes).

My attempts at building a bridge between Eastern and Western thought clearly start from a Western psychological perspective, because I am trying to address Western minds. Some Ayurvedic herbalists, for example, say that in treatment in the West we should be using more Western herbs rather than Indian ones, because of the similar energies between patient and healing medium. In a similar way my book tries to speak to Western minds using the mental concepts (energies) of Western psychological models. However, the underlying practical 'truths' that we will get to are the truths that Sankhya, Ayurveda and yoga have discovered and that inform the spiritual lives of millions around the world.

Ayurveda, the Vedic science of life, is a healing system that is spiritual and holistic in its essence. Ayurveda is thus part of a cosmology that explains the whole of creation and is deeply spiritual in its diagnostic and therapeutic models and practices. It implicitly covers body, mind and soul. The physical, mental and spiritual aspects of disease processes and healing methods cannot be separated in Ayurveda.

According to Ayurveda, the source of all existence is universal Cosmic Consciousness, which manifests as male and female energy. Purusha, often associated with the male energy, is choiceless, passive, pure awareness. Prakruti, the female energy, is active, choiceful consciousness. Both Purusha and Prakruti are eternal, timeless, and immeasurable.[9]

Out of those two cosmic energies, nature manifests down to successively grosser levels of manifestation, ultimately to the levels of inorganic and organic matter including the human body. Mahat (or buddhi in its individual manifestation), is the cosmic intelligence, or the divine mind, that contains all the great principles behind life. Manas is the conditioned mind or sense-mind, which we usually see as the only mind we have. The conditioned mind or sense-mind is sometimes also called the intellect.

Purusha, or pure spirit, is pure consciousness, pure awareness. Ayurveda, and especially Ayurvedic psychology aim at helping us on the way back to Purusha, which happens when we no longer identify with our thoughts and when we can objectively see the entire realm of Prakruti (primordial nature). The main shift that needs to happen in us is that from manas to mahat – from intellect to intelligence, or from conditioned mind to cosmic mind.

Ahamkara (Ego) and Gunas

Ahamkara means 'I-fabrication' and is the process of division and differentiation by which Prakruti and mahat take specific forms. The five senses, five organs of action, and the five elements arise from ahamkara through the three gunas of sattva, rajas and tamas.

> Ego creates the mind and the senses. … Under the influence of ego, the possibility of divergence from nature arises. Prakriti or the natural condition of things can become vikriti – the diseased, disturbed, unnatural or artificial condition. The blindness and attachment caused by the ego is the main cause of spiritual, mental and physical disorders.[10]

We live in a world of extreme splitting and fragmentation at both inner and outer levels. Inner and outer splitting reinforce each other and have created a complex web of separateness and interdependence in our inner and outer worlds. It has become extremely difficult to see the artificial character of ahamkara and thus transcend back to Purusha.

This also means that the chitta nadi, the most important energy channel for the mind, is flowing outwards into the senses instead of inwards into the soul. Many Ayurvedic treatment methods and yoga are about understanding and reversing this process of splitting and fragmentation and the closely connected excessive energy flow into the senses.

The gunas ('what binds') are the basic qualities of primal nature (Prakruti) and are her potential for diversification. Therefore all objects in the world, and we ourselves, are different combinations of the three gunas. Sattva is the quality of stability, harmony and virtue. Rajas is turbulence, passion and activity, and tamas is heavy, dark and dull. The gunas as primal qualities are the energetic origin of the grosser forms of creation like the elements.

The mind is the most subtle form of matter and as such is particularly shaped by the three gunas. The aim of psycho-spiritual development is to increase sattva in the mind as a return to peace and harmony. This is not as simple as it may sound and it depends very much on our starting point, i.e. which guna is predominant in us to start with. If tamas is the predominant mental energy, then rajas will probably initially have to be increased before sattva can become the goal. Ayurveda and yoga offer a wide range of diets, herbs, lifestyles, pranayama and meditation techniques to increase sattva. We shall return to the gunas in Chapter 11.

Changing the Mind

In Vedic and yogic sciences and in Ayurveda, the mind (including the emotions) is regarded as the most subtle form of matter. Therefore positive changes at the level of the mind are most effective in initiating positive changes at the physical level, including our bodies and our actual physical environment. Mind over matter!

But to change our mind is often the most difficult thing to do. Most people go through their lives in ignorance, meaning that they only operate at the most superficial level of conditioned habitual perceptions and ways of thinking about themselves and about the lives they live. They operate more like computers, running the same old software, creating the same old problems, occasionally crashing, and trying the same old inadequate solutions. To then say 'think more positively, give up drinking, love yourself, can't you see?' might occasionally lead to yet another long list of short-lived new year's resolutions. Or it might lead to a life-long struggle of trying to be different, better, more mature, more successful, less anxious, less depressed. The waiting rooms of psychiatric and psychotherapeutic clinics are full of people who indulge in their weekly bit of self-pitying struggle, with the 'help' of 'compassionate' professionals who rely on long-term, regular clients for their careers and their incomes.

This book aims at helping you to 'change your mind', from the sense-mind to the intelligence of the soul. The real solution is to go beyond the superficial level of the mind, to deeper levels of consciousness. There, right inside ourselves is all the wisdom, all the peace and all the bliss that we usually stress ourselves out to find in the world of impermanent, so-called reality. That place inside is written about in the scriptures of the world. Sometimes it is called heaven, sometimes soul, sometimes the super-conscious. It is the place where intellect becomes intelligence, where emotions become feeling, and where attachment becomes devotion to universal truth.

But it is not easy to get to that place. Often it takes a great crisis, an accident, or even a near-death experience to propel people out of their ignorant habitual ways of existing into a deeper way of being. Unfortunately the subconscious part of the mind is so cluttered with layers of stuff that control us that it takes disciplined work to get through to the deeper levels of super-consciousness.

The most important change in your thinking will be to deeply realise a profound paradox: *Your life journey – past, present and future – with all its ups and downs – is your lesson and you only have the rest of your life left to learn the lesson. This puts extreme importance and weight on your actions from now. At the same time the drama of your life is only acting out one tiny but necessary part of the cosmic drama. You are only an actor on a universal stage. Occasionally, just go and sit in the second row and watch the show.*

Throughout this book we will be trying to hold both those perspectives – the excruciating seriousness of the situation and of your actions *and* the fact that your whole life is just a tiny ripple on a gigantic ocean. In practice this means that we will be working on your issues in a serious and disciplined way and that we will also step back from your issues completely so that you can be in the ocean rather than just being the ripple.

> Every man, as it were, is thrown into a boisterous river of the activities of Nature. If he does not swim, if he tries to remain neutral, he will disappear from a world whose keynote is 'Struggle!'. The universal flux does not accommodate a stationary man.[11]

This quote points to something very important. We are part of the struggle of Nature. Where are we in the struggle? Which side are we on? What is the direction, the goal of our very own personal struggle? Which of the forces of nature are we allied with?

Yoga and Ayurveda can give us the models and the tools to analyse and understand universal nature. We need to know the boisterous river, its current, its flow, so that we can find our own direction.

Our world presents to us ready-made goals for our lives. They are usually about more or better objects from the world of matter. Our world lures us to identify with and participate in that part of the struggle of nature that yoga would call illusion because it is wholly associated with gross matter. That way we automatically 'buy' the flip-side of a world of matter which is characterised by duality. By pursuing pleasure, happiness and material gain in the way in which the advocates of materialism in our culture are trying to persuade us to do, we automatically set up experiences of pain, unhappiness and loss for ourselves. One side cannot exist without the other.

> There is a fundamental truth or reality, a state of pure consciousness or pure awareness that is beyond words and thought, in which there is peace, bliss, compassion and liberation. To reach that is the goal of all life.
>
> Life is essentially a state of suffering or unhappiness and this is caused by the ego or principle of selfishness. The ego sets in motion a stream of action or karma, which ties us to a process of rebirth and transmigration in which is repeated sorrow.
>
> To eradicate this suffering it is necessary to negate the ego and silence the mind, as the ego is a function of the mind in its state of disturbance. This

involves going beyond fear, desire and anger, the emotions that keep the mind disturbed.

For this end certain ethical values must be followed like truthfulness, humility and non-violence. For this end the main practice is yoga and meditation. This goal is not a personal goal but part of the liberation of all life and so should be done for the unity and good of all and not just for our personal benefit.[12]

This book tries to help you understand the splitting and fragmentation, and the attachments and addictions that the ego (ahamkara) and the sense-mind (manas) have created. In terms of yoga this book is about pratyahara, which is the withdrawal from wrong food, wrong impressions, wrong associations in order to open up to right food, impressions and associations.

Our commercial society functions by stimulating our interest through the senses. ... The problem is that the senses, like untrained children, have their own will, which is largely instinctual in nature. They tell the mind what to do. If we don't discipline them, they dominate us with their endless demands. ... We run after what is appealing to the senses and forget the higher goals of life. For this reason, pratyahara is probably the most important limb of yoga for people today.[13]

Let us now go on the journey of understanding why and how this is so and how we can go beyond our mental conditioning.

3

Craving Certainty – Addicted to Conflict

This is the world we live in: we feel the intense desire for something certain, for freedom from doubt – a kind of deep inner craving for perfection (craving comes from the Old English *crafian*, which means to beg). But with our senses we experience conflict, disharmony all around us and within. And, let's be honest, there is this part of us that thrives on battles and clashes, even if only in a spectator way. We might call it drama, or news, or 'a good plot'. But conflict it is. Life without conflict would be boring, wouldn't it? To be 'bored stiff' is like being dead. Excitement, entertainment, having a good time, making the most of life, enjoy-ment are all terms that seem to point at the senses, at things out there. The drama of life; living life to the full. None of that seems to go very easily with going inside, to the point of stillness within. We are so used to 'noise'; stillness feels abnormal, even boring.

This, in a way, goes right to the heart of our journey, because a journey it is. The only way out is in implies that getting out is a good thing, but that there is a paradox, that in order to get out we need to go inside. You may have tried several ways of going inside and of getting out. Have any of those ways ever involved trying to go inside to that inner place of stillness and peace, to your inner sanctuary? Well, that's where we're going to go. It is not going to be easy – much easier to rush into yet another corner of the sensual world of multitudes of conflict in search of a certainty that never materialises.

Certainty or 'Trying to be perfect the wrong way'

Richard was referred to me for psychotherapy. Yet another highly qualified, middle aged, senior middle manager whose so-called psychological problems apparently were preventing him from progressing his career further. Richard was a physicist by training and had progressed to managing fifty other scientists in a commercial research establishment. He was finding his leadership role increasingly difficult and periods of depression, irritability and stress were becoming more intense. We spent about ten sessions together figuring out the reasons for his dilemma. It became very clear why Richard was suffering so much in his role. He turned out to be what is commonly labelled 'a perfectionist'. He never liked uncertainties, and his life-story contained, amongst other elements, long formative years at boarding school and a father who constantly and openly worried about things that could go wrong, i.e. just about everything. In his job, those above him and those below him expected Richard to project *certainty*. This worried him a lot. He wanted to appear certain and decisive in his management decisions. His inability to do so, especially when it involved decisions about staff, i.e. real people, appeared to him like a personal failure. This made him worry even more, just like his father. He did not want to be like his father at all. When he was sent to me for psychotherapy he knew that something must be badly wrong with him. A few other counsellors had already tried their skills on him without much success. Maybe he just wasn't 'management material'.

So, was the aim to teach Richard to appear certain, to let go of the legacy of his father, to let go of the deep insecurities of his childhood that were still operating in the adult? Of course there is value in teaching someone to function better, helping them to deal better with their work, their relationships. But on what basis, in what context? What does Richard's dilemma say about the way in which we approach life?

Let us, just for a moment, look at the world as it is, not as we would like it to be. This world is uncertain, and to a large extent unpredictable. Any truth that we have discovered and are discovering is relative and never the total truth. We know very little and we will continue to know little, but our knowledge will also expand if we allow it to expand. But in order for that expansion to happen we need to keep an 'open mind', because chances are that many of today's truths will be untruths in future. We need to be able to face the 'unknown' in most areas of our lives.

The history of science is littered with the corpses of 'hard facts' which have had to give way to newer 'hard facts' as new discoveries were made. What we know about ourselves and nature and the universe is almost certainly greatly outweighed by what we do not know. As Karl Popper put it, our knowledge is always finite, but our ignorance is always infinite. It is surely reasonable to believe that human knowledge will continue to grow so long as there are human beings around to make discoveries and to think. Having said this, it is important that we make provision for the growth of knowledge. One way of doing this is to ensure that we have concepts in which there is room to grow. Our concepts can only ever be as clear and useful as we are capable of making them. However, our capacity to conceive is capable of growth. As it grows, there is a corresponding growth in that which we can conceive and comprehend. If you like, a little more of the depth, richness, mystery and complexity of the world becomes available to us. Yet we can be sure that however much we understand anything today, our understanding will be different in the future. Much of what we are convinced is true today will be replaced by broader, deeper, more accurate knowledge. This should help to put our current knowledge into its proper perspective. We are all familiar with the amused astonishment we feel when we look back and recollect how limited our understanding of something was in the past compared to our current understanding of the same thing. We would do well to recognise that the same process operates forward in time as well as backwards. Our current understanding of anything, which we may well feel to be adequate if not complete today, will almost certainly come to be regarded in time with the same amused astonishment with which we regard our past efforts. Humility is in order as well as excitement when considering our achievements.[14]

Could it be that somewhere deep inside Richard knows this? That somewhere deep inside he does not want to play the game of certainty that has become such a necessity in the world of commerce?

Richard's world is dominated by our longing for certainty and absolute truth and by our belief that we can get it through the acquisition of goods, through jobs, partners. As a manager Richard is expected to feed that need for the sake of the products his company sells and for the sake of the employees who work for him. The more truthful alternative approach would be quite unacceptable in Richard's world. Imagine a manager standing up and saying to his staff and to his firm's customers: 'Look, I am not quite sure about what we are doing at the moment. I think it's ok, but it might not be. Our products are quite safe, as far as we can determine at present. But it might turn out in future that they are carcinogenic or causing some other damage. Our jobs are relatively secure, but with the present uncertainty in the world's financial markets … Who knows?'

People do not want to hear this from their bosses or from their politicians. People want certainties. Political elections are being fought with optimistic messages. Certainties are being produced and sold to customers who want just that. Our longing for those absolute truths, for those absolute certainties is so deep and so strong that the market for certainties is inexhaustible. We want security, certainty, strength, eternal wealth and happiness. And the people who sell us our world, the advertising industry and other brainwashers, fool us into believing that they can satisfy our longing. But that longing is the soul's longing. It is the soul knowing and remembering that absolute truth and certainty do exist somewhere deep inside. Unfortunately we have lost contact with our soul. We have forgotten that those soul qualities cannot exist in the material world. And this is big business. Having forgotten that our craving for certainty and predictability is the soul's craving, we project the need for it onto objects and people – parents, bosses, partners, friends, houses, careers etc.

So, is Richard so wrong, so abnormal, so damaged, when he does not want to play the game? It's quite a difficult question and part of me does not want to take the risk of giving the answer that my elaboration requires. It is risky, because where does it leave psychotherapy and psychotherapists, who have made it their business to feed into the illusion that some kind of blissful state of certainty can be achieved as a result of the tools of their trade? The risky answer then is that Richard's conflict is normal and that it really is a conflict between soul and ego that cannot be adequately resolved by the ego-strengthening techniques of psychotherapy. But then, Richard is a scientist and does not believe in soul and spirit.

As you can possibly gather by now, we are dealing with delicate stuff here. We are dealing with widening the context for our ways of thinking and approaching our lives. In order to widen the context we need to stretch and even break old boundaries and limitations. This is not comfortable, because it creates – guess what? *Uncertainty*!

For our normal everyday mind, uncertainty creates fear and we are convinced that fear needs to be avoided. Whole industries exist just to lull us into the illusion of fearlessness. At the same time fearlessness is mentioned in the *Bhagavad Gita* as 'the impregnable rock on which the house of spiritual life must be erected'.[15] But this is the fearlessness of the soul, a state that the ego can never achieve.

Conflict – or 'the world is in a mess'

We probably all agree with this heading most of the time, because we all feel uncomfortable with so many things. We feel stressed, burnt out, and the media are bashing us with a constant flow of stories about *conflict*. It seems as though conflict makes the world go round. Just spend a few moments trying to remember when you last heard a news story that did not relate to some conflict or other. When did you last watch a TV programme where conflict was not the main theme? How often does conflict provide the topic for our discussions? What do we talk about when there is no conflict? There are so many conflicts – between rich and poor, north and south, men and women, this political party and that, ecologists and non-ecologists, socialism and capitalism and so on, and so on. Newspapers, TV, and especially radio talk-shows thrive on it. Opinions are expressed, contradicted, argued. Strong thoughts and feelings are aroused and expressed or repressed. '*I* am right, you're wrong' and '*I* need everybody else to know that too' is taking up a lot of mental energy in people. And sometimes conflict spills over into action. Wars are being fought, crimes are being committed, lives are being wasted in conflict and battles.

It would not be difficult to imagine that some very sensitive, observant aliens would quickly come to the conclusion that conflict is the psychological fuel that keeps us Earthlings going. We appear to be almost addicted to it. But doesn't this contradict our deep but unacknowledged craving for peace, certainty, permanence and perfection?

There obviously is a contradiction if we look at it the way we are used to looking at it. But let us try to widen the context again, as we did with Richard and his struggle with certainty. Both our need for certainty and our attachment to conflict are big business. The marketing and selling of cars can serve as an example. They are usually marketed with both elements. The shape, brand, colour and other aspects can suggest certainty, solidity, permanence, security, reliability. In addition there are elements that speak to our need for conflict, competition, being better, faster, safer, stronger than the other brands on the market.

The skill in marketing and selling seems to be to address both human needs concurrently. In addition, the apparent contradiction between certainty and conflict allows for further business strategies. TV news, the main forum for conflict stories, are usually read by the same newsreaders who appear fatherly or motherly, or at least solid and serious, thus giving the impression of consistency and certainty. The same is true for radio talk-show hosts – same time, same voice, first names. Conflict is made safe. On the other hand, products that represent solidity and certainty are often advertised in a highly charged, competitive environment, containing elements of conflict.

What we lose sight of in all this is the fact that certainty is a soul-quality, while conflict is a characteristic of the world of matter. If we look at it like this, the whole story changes. We find that our culture has turned soul qualities of certainty (truth) and permanence (eternity) into marketing tools. We are led to believe that we can buy states of mind that used to be the province of religion and spirituality. We are also led to believe that the qualities of matter are at least equal to the qualities of the soul, because both appear to be connected with objects.

This is not so. According to the Vedas what we perceive as reality is not. What we perceive is *only* the world of matter which is based in the principle of duality, and which ultimately is an illusion that we can transcend. On the basis of this hypothesis I should therefore like to encourage you to *trust* your unease with the world as it seems to be. Later on we shall explore the psychological and social mechanisms that create this internal and external world of duality and conflict. Through this exploration we shall then touch that place of certainty and unity that we all carry inside us and which is called soul.

Introduction to Reflections and Exercises

This is the first reflection in this book. First of all I should like to introduce the purpose and format of the reflections and exercises to you. All the reflections aim at deepening and personalising what you have read so far. You can either do or not do the reflections. It is entirely up to you. You may just want to read through the book and then come back to the reflections and exercises later. Or you may want to do them as a group exercise. The reflections and exercises are your personal space. Use the space wisely and in a way that is appropriate for you.

All the reflections and exercises are meditations. They are trying to help you develop the habit of meditating regularly. Proper meditation is about clearing the mind, or going beyond our thinking. The reflections will guide you gradually to this point by first of all involving your thinking in a way that is different from your usual way. However, it will be useful if you take on a meditative body posture for the reflections right away.

You can do the reflections and exercises in either a sitting or lying position. Meditation is usually practised in a sitting position.

IDEAL SITTING POSITION

The best and most comfortable position for relaxation and meditation is to sit upright with your back and head as straight as possible without tension. Pull your shoulders back slightly and push your chest out a bit. Put your chin up a little. Have your hands on your lap with your palms facing up or with one hand cupped in the other. Have your legs uncrossed and be aware of the contact of your feet with the ground. But most importantly, the position must not cause tension or pain. If you are a 'sloucher', you could take up the ideal position and then slouch back to your normal position. Somewhere in between will be right for you. Stretching and movement exercises, like those taught in yoga classes, are ideal to prepare your body for a good meditation posture.

IDEAL LYING POSITION

Lie on your back with your head on a small cushion or pillow to keep your neck as straight as possible. Have your arms by your side preferably with your palms facing up. Have your legs next to one another with your feet falling out slightly. Make sure you are comfortable. If you have a lower back problem you might find it helpful to have a cushion under your knees. Use a blanket if you cannot keep warm otherwise.

OTHER PRELIMINARIES

It is best to have your eyes closed for each exercise. If you find that difficult, you may want to start off with your eyes half closed.

While doing the exercises you may have all sorts of unrelated thoughts come into your mind. Don't fight them or get angry with yourself. Just acknowledge those interfering thoughts and let them go.

CONFLICT AND FEAR (REFLECTION 1)

1. Spend a few moments reflecting on what certainty and conflict mean for you.
Remember times in your life when you felt very certain about yourself, or a situation, or your life, or your future. What was it like to feel like that? Where in your body did you feel it? How long did the certainty last?

Remember situations in your life when you were thriving on conflict. Which emotions were dominant for you then? Excitement, anger, joy? Where in your body did you feel those feel-

ings? How did you feel when the conflict was over?

2. Now look back over your life and see what role fear has played in your life. How is fear keeping you stuck? What have you been afraid of? What would need to happen for you to let go of your fear?

3. Read the following poem and reflect on it for a few minutes with your eyes closed.

The Choice for Love

What does the voice of fear
whisper to you?

Fear speaks to you
in logic and reason.
It assumes the language
of love itself.

Fear tells you,
'I want to make you safe.'
Love says,
'You are safe.'

Fear says,
'Give me symbols.
Give me frozen images.
Give me something
I can rely on.'

Loving truth says,
'Only give me
this moment.'

Fear would walk you
on a narrow path
promising to take you
where you want to go.

Love says,
'Open your arms
and fly with me.'

Every moment of your life
you are offered the opportunity
to choose –
love or fear,
to tread the earth
or to soar the heavens.[16]

4

Changing Your Mind

Overstimulation of the Senses

*H*arry had had enough. Everything was getting too much for him – work, family, mortgage, the whole lot. Life had become an endless struggle, and the old distractions, sex
and alcohol, didn't work any more either. Panic attacks, depression, binge-drinking, and
eventually Prozac and psychotherapy. Harry now knew how he was handicapped in the
area of forming mature attachments. The insights gained in psychotherapy helped Harry
a great deal – he felt more grown-up, more mature. But still – something was missing in
Harry's life. He still wasn't happy, and he felt he should be now that he had done so much
work on himself.

Our world is teaching us to expect complete happiness and fulfilment in this
life-time. The way to get it seems to be 'out there' in all the things we have created,
and can purchase or achieve. But then we can still find ourselves 'on the edge',
when we have struggled and fought to achieve that blissful state that advertising,
education, and even medicine and psychotherapy promise us. When we have put
all our energy into our careers, families, possessions and we are still unhappy, then
we begin to ask the 'big questions' – the questions about the meaning of life and
death, *our* life and *our* death.

We are bombarded with stimulation and temptation of the senses. According
to the Henley Centre's Media Futures Report we were exposed to 1300 commercial messages each day in 1997. In total there were 11,000 television adverts
broadcast every day in 1997, compared with 1987 when there were 500 shown a
day.[17]

This 'overstimulation' of the senses by man-made objects and messages has
gone hand-in-hand with a disconnection from the natural world, which is
degraded to a thing to be exploited. Surrounded by the objects of our desires like
an impenetrable wall, we have lost contact with the spiritual energies of God and
the Earth (Heavenly Father and Divine Mother).

We are becoming uncomfortable with this situation. Something feels not quite
right. Depression, obsession, addiction are the expressions of the suffering that
descends like a dark hang-over after too much bingeing.

Increasing numbers of people are looking for, or are forced to look for, meaning in their lives beyond the promise of bliss through yet more purchases, bigger houses, better careers, clothes, wives, husbands, families. The 'bigger better more faster' culture is driving our intra- and inter-personal structures to breaking point. Emotional and physical crises are the obvious results, and psychiatry and even psychotherapy try to fix things through pills and *personal growth*.

Psychotherapy

Whilst both pills and personal growth can help, and are often essential to soften or shift some of the inner emotional blocks and conflicts that have been there for a long time, they must not be confused with a 'spiritual path'. The pills, usually anti-depressants or tranquillisers, do not suit some people, can have severe so-called side-effects, and can be addictive. Certain psychotherapies, even though they are a form of 'going inside', can be very expensive and time consuming and can create in us a view of ourselves and the world (a mindset) that can ultimately even distract from a spiritual path as advocated here. Other approaches are different, and 'psychosynthesis', for example, even includes spiritual elements in its models and approach. However, some of the dangers still persist. The reason probably is that however inspired a model or a technique might initially be, as human beings we always have the potential to infuse it with the desires and attachments of the ego (power, greed, envy), as long as the model does not specifically and strongly guard against this.

For example, you might feel tired and have a headache when you arrive late for your session with your psychotherapist, because you got stuck in several major traffic jams, your car does not have air-conditioning, it was a very hot day, and your head aches from the car fumes that you had to breathe in. Your therapist may well interpret your angry complaints about the terrible journey as your 'resistance', or as your rage against him, which is basically seen as your infantile rage against your mother or your father, and which you are not expressing appropriately – as yet. He may well say something like: 'I don't want to doubt that the journey was really difficult. But I can't help wondering whether the external conditions of your journey somehow reflect the inner struggle you have about becoming really engaged in your therapy.' Your spiritual counsellor, on the other hand, would probably be more likely to invite you to meditate with him, so that you could distance yourself from the journey and re-charge with life energy.

Another example would be when you tell your psychotherapist that you've found these spiritual teachings and you want to follow them and you've reached a stage where the connection with 'Divine Mother' is becoming more important than your early childhood issues with your real mother. Chances are that your psychotherapist will see that as your defence against 'really working on your issues'. He will probably see your wish as yet another expression of your resistance or defence against some deeply unconscious rage that you are holding against him (in transference). Psychoanalysis always has the potential of promoting the ego to a god-like state, which can then only be perfected by spending many years of wading through the mud of the subconscious mind.

An American psychiatrist describes how psychiatry would view the attempt to distance oneself from the world of matter and duality, which usually is part of a spiritual path:

> Psychiatry's position is that to try to become unaffected by such a central system in our lives [the system of duality – RK] is in fact a defensive measure, a way to repress or deny our true identity. Psychiatrists for the most part do not believe that there is a higher self or a level of consciousness beyond duality. Their position is that God is manufactured by man; belief in a higher self is a defence against emotions. On the other hand is the spiritual attitude: attachment to the emotions is a defence against realizing one's higher self.[18]

I am sure that some of my psychotherapist colleagues will criticise me for my views. They might say that I am just expressing my unresolved anger about my profession, and ultimately my parents (unresolved transference). I should have stayed in psychotherapy longer, they will say. But after fifteen years on the receiving and giving end of psychotherapy, I am beginning to doubt the universal truth of these 'elegant' interpretations.

However, there may well be some 'higher truth' in psychological and psychoanalytical models. We shall in later chapters explore some of those truths in some of the models. After all, the 'laws of nature' that we have been and are discovering, be they psychological or physical, are all part of universal truth. In this context it is interesting to note that Freudian psychology has identified the oedipal conflict of separation from father and wanting to merge with mother as the root of modern psychopathology. Could this, at a 'higher level', represent the inter-personal and intra-psychic expression of our spiritual separation from Heaven and Earth? Even many of the Freudian concepts – defence mechanisms, object relations and splitting, and projection – may well express and reflect parallel global or collective processes of surrounding ourselves with multitude, complexity and fragmentation, and then having to project our deprived divinity (loss of connection with Heaven and Earth) onto poor man-made substitutes.

The approach taken throughout this book is that our *crises* also present our opportunity to hear the soul's craving for a spiritual path. In this context we will use psychological models as maps, just as I use them in my work with myself and with my clients, because our knowledge, our *truths* are never completely wrong. The laws that we have discovered, the laws out of which we have created aeroplanes, computers, space exploration, medicine, psychology, are not wrong. But they can never be the whole truth; they are not religion. They can become destructive only when we try to promote them to total truths.

What is needed is a radically different approach to ourselves, our lives and our world. In order to get out of the rat-race we need to go inside to that inner point of stillness, to our soul. From that point we can become co-creators in the vast process of creation. We can operate in a soul-directed rather than a sense-directed way. From that point within we can even create the world we want.

Holy, Holistic and Holographic

Apart from getting away from the over-stimulation of the senses, a move that is advocated by most of the world's religions, there is another, not so immediately obvious but connected purpose to this 'going-inside' business. We are all one at many different levels, but we are faced with a world that is amazingly fragmented. Boundaries and separation are the issues that surround us, whereas underneath we are all connected with one another and with everything. The only way for us to see reality as it really is, is by going inside ourselves; otherwise we will remain stuck in fragmentation and ultimately suffering.

This notion of our ultimate inter-connectedness and one-ness with the universe and beyond is not coming out of some mystical, new-age belief, but is arising out of two areas of science – quantum theory and cosmology. Physicists like Bohm, who has been exploring the behaviour of the smallest known particles, and mathematician and cosmologist Brian Swimme, who is investigating and telling the story of the universe, are presenting us with findings that turn our established view of reality upside down.

You may think that quantum theory and cosmology are really not your 'cup of tea'. But all around us, including in the world of science, connections between different areas of science and our psychological and spiritual paths are emerging. We need to look and see. Now, for the first time in history as we know it, we have come full circle. We have reached a point where the teachings of the ancient Indian masters are being substantiated by the latest discoveries and considerations of Western science. We are asked to let go of our well established views of reality. Our consciousness is urged to make the 'quantum leap' of seeing ourselves as part of the whole and the whole as part of ourselves. It is a big challenge, but it is also increasingly becoming a life and death issue for many individuals and for humanity as a whole. The universe is awaiting us to embrace our destiny.

We live in this world of conflicts and contradictions, suffering the passing of time, and ultimately death. Our rational, 'down to earth' friends say, that's how it is and that's all there is. We're just a bundle of cells, having 'evolved' by trial and error out of some general soup of organic life, which itself has evolved out of some soup of inorganic life. They claim that even consciousness can be explained in terms of natural laws and therefore is a function of matter. So what? Just because we have discovered certain laws and can see those laws operating in the things we observe and measure, does not mean that is all there is to it. It is like the old dispute in psychology/psychiatry whether depression is functional (i.e. psychological) or biological in origin. Having taken part in many disputes like this over the years, I now find them so futile. Of course, depression is both psychological and biological. It just depends how, from what angle, with what measuring instruments you look at it. All human behaviour is always psychological and biological. But both systems of knowledge, psychology and biology, are man-made and are therefore likely to be superseded by different models, systems, measuring instruments etc. in future. Just because we can explain a lot by using the laws we have discovered and by using the models and instruments we have developed, does not mean that there are not laws behind the laws behind the laws and so forth.

The new discoveries in quantum physics and in cosmology are now beginning to make it possible to argue against our rational friends, using rational arguments without having to rely entirely on vague mysticism, faith and devotion and thereby running the risk of being dismissed by our friends as esoteric 'weirdos'.

Science is discovering and beginning to tell the story of mystery. Spirit is beginning to reveal itself all around us, cutting through our solid layers of scientific 'rationality'. I am talking here about the inter-connectedness of everything. It is such an enormous thing to grasp. But once you grasp it, once you begin to see it, it is immensely re-assuring and exciting. And then you begin to see, hear and sense messages and connections everywhere. This is also the message that Redwood puts across in *The Celestine Prophecy*.[19] Eventually you begin to ask what the underlying theme of all those connected messages might be. Then it becomes very difficult to not end up with an affirmation of God and Spirit.

I have mentioned the quantum vacuum earlier. It basically says that space is not empty, and that all the solid things we see and feel are just stationary waves. Just imagine – trees and all matter are stationary waves in the zero-field of the quantum vacuum. Light, consciousness and energy are just different waves in the same field. I shall let two representatives of the new science movement express their views in their own words. Irvin Laszlo, systems philosopher and founder of the Club of Budapest writes about the zero-field:

> What fills the whole of space is an intense energy known as 'zero-point field'. In itself, this vast field is not electromagnetic, gravitational, or nuclear. Instead, it is the originating source, not only of all these known fields, but also of the matter particles themselves. The energy density of the zero-point field is well-nigh inconceivable. ... We are fortunate that this stupendous energy does not impinge on our world in the same way as the positive energy we know. This is because it is what physicists call 'virtual' or negative energy. When sufficiently destabilized, however, a region of the zero-point field can be kicked from negative into positive, and so give rise to matter. This is what is thought to have happened in the Big Bang, when the observable universe was created. But, once created, matter maintains close connections with the

vacuum field, in the form of the inertial force. ... Thus all the fundamental characteristics we normally associate with matter are vacuum interaction products: inertia, mass, as well as gravity. In the emerging concept there is no 'absolute matter', only an absolute matter-generating energy field. Although this view of matter and space seems to turn things upside down, in some way it appeals more to common-sense than do the standard conceptions of 20th century physics. After all, if light is a wave, then something should be waving. This is space-time, which can now claim the status of a physical reality. Light and sound are travelling waves in this continuous energy field, and tables and trees, rocks and swallows, and other seemingly solid objects are standing waves in it.[20]

And here Brian Swimme ponders the implications of this new view of reality:

If material stuff is understood to be the very foundation of being, we are quite naturally going to devote our lives and education to the task of acquiring such stuff, for human beings have an innate tropism for being. ... Just as an earlier age devoted itself to serving the dictates of the kings in order to become involved with the really real, so too does our age dedicate itself to acquiring commodities in order to enter the wonderworld promised by our advertisers. ...

The appropriation of the new cosmology depends upon an understanding of the reality and power of the nonvisible and nonmaterial realm. ...

Each particular thing is directly, and essentially, grounded in all-nourishing abyss. Though we think of our bodies as dense and completely filling up the space they occupy, careful investigation of matter has shown that this is not the case. The volume of elementary particles is extremely small when compared to the volume of the atoms they form. Thus, the essential nature of any atom is less material than it is 'empty space'. Even from this elementary perspective we can begin to appreciate that the root foundation of any thing or any being is not the matter out of which it is composed so much as the matter together with the power that gives rise to the matter. ...

In the next millennium, young people educated in the new cosmology will experience the Moon not as a frozen lump but as an event that trembles into existence each moment. Moonlight will be understood not as bounced from the Sun but as expressive of the Moon's reality. They will regard the Moon not as dead object but as a creative source, as an origin of the universe, a geyser in the sky where the universe sprays into existence.

Through such encounters we learn that the universe is not a collection of dead objects but is, rather, a seamless whole community made up of cosmos-creating subjects.[21]

Recently scientists pondering why life could develop and be maintained on Earth in comparison to Mars or Venus, discovered the important role that processes have that at first sight appear threatening to life. In part life on Earth is maintained by the constant re-cycling of carbon dioxide, which is 'frozen' in rocks on Mars and dispersed in the hot atmosphere on Venus. On Earth the carbon dioxide gets washed out of the atmosphere by rain and is then caught in rocks. But the process does not stop there. The movement of the tectonic plates, causing earthquakes, pulls the rocks into the hot interior of the Earth, from where the carbon-dioxide then gets released again into the atmosphere through the eruption of volcanoes. What a wonderfully complex and circular process, where creation and destruction interact in the building of the conditions for life.

Paramahansa Yogananda frequently uses the metaphor of the wave and the sea. We and everything else in this world of matter are just waves and ripples on the vast ocean of God's cosmic dream. Our individual soul is like a wave on the vast ocean of spirit. Rippled by the wind, the wave is never really disconnected from the sea. And after its brief existence it returns to be part of the ocean again.

As [the gunas] move across the Ocean of Infinity, individualized waves are whipped into being. The large waves, swept farthest from the quiet oceanic depths, are the waves of evil, those lives most affected by the storm of delusion. The medium waves are the active lives, surging along in Nature's ebb and flow. The small waves of good lives remain closest to the Ocean's bosom, buffeted the least by the prevailing winds of change.[22]

The Vedic Sankhya system (see Chapter 2) states that behind the world of matter, driving and creating it, there is spirit, consisting of energy, emptiness, thought, ideas. Vedic philosophy and Ayurvedic medicine and psychology contain complex models explaining all the inter-connections between the different levels of energies and matter. Western science too is beginning to discover that the world of matter that we experience as solid and real is largely made up of light and sound and is not nearly as solid as we think.

Love and Knowledge (Heart and Mind)

Many people want to get out – out of the rat-race, out of poverty, out of cities, suffering, neuroses etc. 'Getting away from it all' dominates whole industries. People want to live in the countryside. They commute into the cities creating stress, pollution. Countryside homes in commutable distance from cities are becoming more expensive. People need to work more, earn more, pollute more in order to be able to afford their home in the country. And so it goes on.

Our world is dominated by 'externality'. We look for bliss, happiness, satisfaction outside ourselves. We're looking the wrong way, because we can only really find it if we look inside. Only there can we connect with our centre that is the centre of the universe and with the energy that is behind all objects. But we do not know how to look inside any more. It's almost as though we've forgotten that there is something inside ourselves – our Self, our soul, God. And it's not surprising that we've forgotten – there are so many other things to occupy our minds, to keep us busy.

The way out of our suffering is to go inside. It's a paradox, but it is something where all the religions of the world agree. The key is reflection and meditation.

But first of all we need to calm down our mind. There is no point in just saying 'OK, I'll meditate then.' Our mind will soon find many reasons why this is utterly impractical and a waste of time. We can and usually will find better things to do. Vivekananda, an Indian Swami who came to the West around the turn of the last century, says that ideally we should have a strong mind connected with a strong heart:

> What is now wanted is a combination of the greatest heart with the highest intellectuality, of infinite love with infinite knowledge. ... Existence without Knowledge and Love cannot be; Knowledge without Love, and Love without Knowledge cannot be.[23]

So we first of all need to convince the mind, our intellect, that this 'going inside' might be a good idea. That does not mean that the mind will not rebel against the whole project later on. But by gently convincing the mind we will get some breathing space (space for the breath) in which we can build soul-strength. Then the battle proper can start – the inner battle between good and evil, between good habits and bad habits. Battle sounds a bit bombastic and perhaps frightening. But a battle it is, very much like the one on the plains of Kurukshetra, as described in the *Bhagavad Gita*.

The goal is quite clear – Self-realisation or the soul's journey back to God (from where it comes in the first place). Your Western, rational, logical mind might be rebelling against words like religion, soul, Self, Hindu, Bhagavad Gita etc., because all you really want to know is how to make things better for yourself.

I am saying that, at this stage, you don't know how bad things really are. You don't really have the tools to examine your existence, your being, your life and your death. Our culture is not giving you the words, the concepts to see and experience yourself within the context of the whole universe. This book is trying to give you the tools to assess your life and to change the way you see it and ultimately the way you lead it.

We are just beginning to think of planet Earth, of humanity, as a whole unit. But concepts like quantum vacuum are not commonplace yet. To grasp life, time, space, i.e. 'the lot', as a whole with you in it, and it in you – that's a different story altogether. We are not used to thinking like that. Your mother didn't, your father didn't, your teachers probably didn't. So why should you?

And here I am, promising you some obscure battle for self-realisation. No wonder that your mind, your intellect are rebelling. You want peace of mind and an easy life. You want to harvest the fruits of your struggles – nice house, nice car, nice partner, nice children etc. Happiness, bliss is what you want and you want the easiest way of getting it. You deserve it, don't you?

But there also is a different voice in you. A voice that speaks quite a different language. That voice speaks a strange language. It's the voice behind your neuroses, your addictions, your frustrations, your crises. It's the voice that tries to speak to you when you feel very lonely, when you're down, when you feel there is no point. You might want to drown that voice, distract from it, but it comes back, again and again. Your body and your ego translate that voice into anxiety, depression and despair. I am saying: listen to that voice differently, try to understand what it is saying. Maybe there is a translation problem.

What you know is that there is this rather annoying part of you that comes out in the most uncomfortable ways at the most inconvenient times. It's becoming more difficult to run away from it. The anti-depressants and the tranquillisers may have helped for a while, but it's still coming back – at night, first thing in the morning, or when your mind isn't busy with other things. Can you hear the yearning, the longing in that little voice behind the emotional turmoil? That little voice is the soul trying to speak in that gentle tone that you have forgotten how to understand. Your body and your emotions are frightened of that voice, because they know it could herald the beginning of the end of their dominance over your life. That little voice has the innocence of a child. It is a calm, wise child that is quietly pleading with you – the soul-child or Christ-child that we all carry in our hearts and in our minds.

On these pages I am asking your mind to hear and understand that voice. I am writing to your mind to listen to your soul-voice so that what you really are deep down inside can emerge and relieve you from the suffering of misunderstandings, misinterpretations, conflicts and crises – in short, from what the Hindus call maya.

The way I am doing it here is by addressing your mind, knowing that there is a deeper (or higher) part of your mind, the intuitive mind, that can go beyond where your rational mind has led you. But this does not mean that we are neglecting or demeaning rationality. Rationality just needs to be 'held' in the wider context of your intuition or your heart.

I despise the often given pseudo-psychotherapeutic advice that you have to 'get in touch with your feelings' and be 'less mind-controlled'. It is more complicated than this. In Ayurveda the mind holds both thoughts and feelings.

The mind, like the wind blows the clouds of thoughts and feelings. Yet the mind is not only like the wind, it is also like space. It encompasses and pervades all its contents, like a screen that holds all the pictures placed upon it. The mind is the most subtle form of matter.[24]

We need to transcend the mind and the feelings that are dominated by external sensations and their resulting thoughts and memories, in order to reach the deeper levels of intelligence and consciousness that are connected with the soul.

The Meaning of Life Question

Sometimes it can happen like this. You might be sitting at home, in the pub, be driving on the motorway – suddenly you find yourself right where you are in your life, and this unfamiliar question runs through your mind: 'How did I get here and why?' Or the question might sound something like: 'What am I doing here?' Your mind may have come up with simpler versions of the question before, but you might have ignored it, or you may have automatically used one of the many ways of distracting from the 'niggles'. But now it's right there, occupying all of you, and you probably wish that the question had never arisen.

When this question is there, all you have left ever to find an answer is the rest of your life, and that remaining rest is becoming smaller by the day, the hour, the minute, the second. So, you should not waste time. There is a certain urgency about it. How and why did I get here and what am I doing here? You may want to try and push it out of your mind, because it is uncomfortable. It would be much easier if the question had not come up in the first place. But now it is there, chances are that the rest of your life will be inter-linked with it. The rest of your life might even depend on it. Depend on it? Why? The answer to this rather bombastic statement will emerge as we go along.

Providing that the old distraction habits like sex, alcohol, TV, shopping, work and children have lost some of their attraction or effectiveness, in order to make sense of that turmoil that has started inside you, possibly even leading to depression and other unpleasant emotions, you might decide to go into psychotherapy. You want to 'work through' your past in order to understand the present. Let us then assume that you find an excellent psychotherapist who knows his/her business. You will probably find out that your past has provided you with many reasons for having ended up neurotic, depressed, narcissistic etc. You then get excited: 'I can work it out!'

That initial flash of hope that things can be 'worked on' and might even get better, is brilliant. Counselling and psychotherapy depend on it. Suddenly you have your one hour per week (at least) when you 'work on your stuff'. One hour of sanity, hope, acceptance, movement, development. There are so many fascinating, exciting, complex models and experiences – your mind is becoming engrossed in understanding how your present miseries have culminated in the 'big question' and were triggered by past trauma, possibly even as far back as past lives (if your therapist is into that). From now on it's 'personal growth', your mind says, and soon you may be finding yourself chasing rainbows in the world of personal development. The market place has become enormous. There are so many things you can buy and do. Instead of chasing after computers, careers and cars, you now hunt after crystals and remedies, workshops and deeply meaningful experiences. Addictions can be swapped so easily.

But what has happened to the initial question that you started out with? It probably will have got lost again in the frantic haste of your self-development activities and in the complexities of the models that your mind is eagerly processing. The question came from your soul, or a place pretty close to it. The mind finds soul-messages a bit 'airy-fairy' and does its best to re-define them as 'interesting thoughts'. Add frantic activity to it and the soul-cry can soon turn into yet another passion, addiction, habit etc.

Psychotherapy and the Meaning of Life

Some statement about the meaning of life is implicit in most models of psychotherapy. The assumption is that the alleviation of suffering through a healing process is possible. In behaviourism this healing is achieved through de-conditioning of conditioned learning. In psychoanalysis through reaching a certain maturity by ceasing to be controlled by repressed emotional material that originates in the past. Most other models fall somewhere between these positions. So, it's all about moving on; letting go of the past; making us whole and healthier. But where are we supposed to move on to?

Despite the undoubted numerous healing benefits that it can provide, this is exactly the point where psychotherapy fails us, because it does not tell us where to move on to, once we have let go of the past. It does not offer a sense of future or wider context, other than to achieve 'maturity' or some sense of 'balance' or 'happiness'. Psychotherapy does not go beyond the sense-mind; it tries to help you achieve bliss and happiness within the world of duality. According to yoga and Ayurveda this state of bliss is not possible without going to the soul first.

But in a way it is good that psychotherapy does not automatically prescribe a 'soul-journey', because we are all on different journeys. We have different starting points, different goals. There are similarities in groups of people though. And these similarities then often fool us into trying to find 'rules' that apply to everybody. Research, theories, statistics and politics all aim at dividing the world or things or people up into clearly defined groups and sub-groups according to a particular model or a set of assumptions.

One assumption would be that, because we are all biologically so similar, we must also be mentally and spiritually similar. This is called 'biological determinism' and all the healing models and professions are infested by it. We want to classify and clarify by grouping objects, people, events. We want to create boundaries, so that we can call this 'this', and that 'that'. It's how our mind works; it's how we have learnt to see the world. But through the creation of boundaries we also create opposites and conflicts and, in the case of psychotherapy, end up with certain treatments for specific disorders and complaints. We then take these groupings that we have created for reality and certainty, and forget that they were just our creation in the first place.

For example we can draw the very simplest form of a boundary line as a circle, and see that it discloses an inside versus an outside. But notice that the opposites of inside vs. outside didn't exist in themselves until we drew the boundary of the circle. ... In short, to draw boundaries is to manufacture opposites. Thus we can start to see that the reason we live in a world of opposites is precisely because life as we know it is a process of drawing boundaries.[25]

But each one of us lives in a different life, and only through acknowledging and experiencing this can we join together. Just imagine, a different unique life pattern and task in everybody and all we can ever really know is our very own, mine. This is why psychotherapy cannot tell us where to move on to, once we have processed all 'our stuff'. The notion of our essential alone-ness and ultimate one-ness is complex. If psychotherapy wants to include this gigantic notion, it needs the help of religion.

Like other great ancient civilizations, India never separated science from philosophy and religion. Rather, it viewed all knowledge as part of a whole designed to promote human happiness, health, and growth. Philosophy is the love of truth. Science is the discovery of truth through experiment. Religion is the experience of truth and application of it in daily living.[26]

Hinduism says that all life on Earth is about the soul's journey back to God. But this happens over many lifetimes. We re-incarnate and have many lifetimes for the journey. So, at this point in time, in this world, in this culture we are all at totally different stages of 'the journey of the soul'. There are 'old souls' and 'young souls'. And there are groups of people with great soul similarities.

The questions always have to be, 'What is this soul trying to work out in this lifetime?' and 'Why is this soul part of my path in this life?' These two questions are bigger than the scientific one of 'who is this individual, which group does he fit into?', or the psychological one of 'what is the transference in this relationship?'. The latter are personality questions, whereas the former are soul questions. Soul-orientated psychotherapy would therefore try to see how the soul's struggle to get back to God is reflected in the life pattern of each individual. It will see the soul at different stages of the battle with the ego, e.g. the battle on the holy plain of Kurukshetra in the *Bhagavad Gita*, or the Six Realms in Buddhist teachings.

Buddhist and Hindu approaches offer methods of speeding up the journey of the soul. The methods all revolve around meditation. Meditation is a way of going inside in order to go beyond the limitations of our life in the world of matter. It's a paradox: less in order to get more; separating and going inside in order to connect with the whole; stillness in order to hear the cosmic sound.

I am sure that personal psychotherapy can help remove the emotional blocks that drain so much physical and mental energy, and thus free the path to the inner sanctuary. But psychotherapy itself is *not* the path. And, unfortunately, for some of us the battle will not lead all the way to soul victory in this life. So I, as a psychotherapist or teacher, need to know what my lesson is, and where my inner battlefield is. I need to own my personality struggle plus the soul struggle that is reflected in it. I can then attract souls who need to reach my level (part) of the struggle. Difficulties can arise with psychotherapists who do not have a soul perspective. Let us briefly consider the example of *attachments*. Psychotherapies are full of theories about right attachments or mature attachments. Spiritual teachings are full of letting go of all attachments. Many spiritual Masters left their family attachments behind. So how does the psychotherapist deal with someone who does not seem to be able or willing to form an attachment with another person? Is it a neurotic deficiency or the sign of a spiritual quest? It is certainly not easy to answer this question, but it is important that both possibilities are considered. Otherwise it can become very easy to see a genuine soul-craving as a neurotic liability.

All this sounds a bit bombastic, doesn't it? Criticisms of anything, in this case the limitations of psychotherapy, are dangerous because they again form groups of 'this is right' and 'that is wrong'. But then, even the use of words in itself creates groups and boundaries. That is why Yogananda says that we should focus on the spirit behind the words when we read inspirational or sacred texts. It is like reading with the heart, or understanding with the intuitive mind rather than with the rational mind.

Later on we shall explore the psychological and sociological dynamics through which we divide the world up into chunks that the intellectual mind can digest.

Chasing Rainbows (Maya)

Spiritual knowledge is the only thing that can destroy our miseries for ever; any other knowledge removes wants only for a time. It is only with the knowledge of the Spirit that the root cause of want is destroyed for ever; so helping man spiritually is the highest help that can be given him. He who gives man spiritual knowledge is the greatest benefactor of mankind, and we always find that they are the most powerful who help man in his spiritual needs, because spirituality is the true inspiration of all our activities. A spiritually strong and sound man will be strong in every other respect, if he so wishes. Until there is spiritual strength in a man, even physical needs cannot be well satisfied.[27]

How true this statement is. I think of those many patients who come to me for psychotherapy with their frustrated needs for perfection. As we shall see later, most so-called 'neurotic' conditions are based in the frustrated need for perfection. If I could only be less shy, less anxious, more socially skilled, more efficient, less depressed, better in relationships, then things, my life, could be perfect or, at least, better. All the different psychotherapies and personal development approaches play into this philosophy – removing a block here, maturing a bit there, improving, relaxing, growing, leaving the past behind etc. They can all feed into the 'bliss illusion'.

So, Vivekananda, the great Hindu master, says that the only knowledge that can get us out of the rut is spiritual knowledge. In this respect, I think, psychotherapy often does work, because there are many spiritual elements in psychotherapy; and it is those elements that further the patient's spiritual path, that do the healing.

... worldly people are seldom impressed by stories of the saints who have worn sackcloth and lived in seclusion. 'What lives of foolish self-denial and misery!' With this airy summing-up, the average man turns his entire attention on the world. To him it appears that happiness must be sought in family life, with its dinner parties, dances, and general stimulation of the senses. The unthinking man does not notice that mankind, busily engaged like himself in chasing the rainbow of lasting happiness, never finds it.[28]

A powerful statement. But isn't this a bit extreme? Can't we find happiness in this life if we do enough work on ourselves? If we spend enough time in therapy, becoming mature, working on our 'stuff', won't we finally reach the state of having a 'fulfilled life'?

No! Because once we do all this work on ourselves, our expectations of what a 'fulfilled life' means, change. At this point in time we might feel that everything will be OK if we just remove this block or that neurosis. But then, once they are removed, we find another layer of different inconsistencies. And so it goes on. It's like peeling an onion (including the tears) – and what is at the core?

Scott-Peck describes how he introduces his work to his new psychotherapy patients.[29] He tells them that he cannot promise them greater happiness as a result of their sessions with him, but what he can promise them is 'greater competence'. Then he adds that there is a catch with this. He says that there seems to be a vacuum of competence in the universe, so that as soon as you are more competent, you get greater problems thrown your way. But, he assures them, their lives will become more interesting.

And as we go on, reaching ever higher levels of competence or awareness, we are faced with greater problems, and then we die. Isn't it like playing a game? We go through life and accumulate increasing levels of complexities – family, career, mortgages, pension plans. We completely lose sight of the simplicity that was there when we were children. Occasionally, on holidays or during those rare special moments, we feel that awesome big feeling – bliss, peace, beauty. We're grateful when it happens. But usually it is only a fleeting moment, a wave that goes through us – free of fear, free of depression, free of worries. Total peace, total harmony, at one with everything. 'That's nice', we think and then it's gone. Our mind continues with its usual busy-ness.

The great Hindu masters say that this feeling is our normal state, our soul-state. But why are we in this normal state so rarely? Why do we have to struggle so hard to achieve brief glimpses of bliss, only to then lose them again and move onto the next struggle?

These questions bring us fairly close to the big question: 'What is the meaning of life?' The other day, the presenter on a talk-radio station put the question to his listeners. About himself he said that he was an agnostic, and didn't believe in after-life or re-incarnation. 'So what can the meaning of life be for agnostics like me?' he asked. One woman sent him a fax, saying 'Please free me from the tyranny of having to ask the question about the meaning of life.' The presenter liked this; he thought it was brilliant. A man phoned in and said that animals knew that life was about having as much joy as possible. Why did we, as human beings have to make it so complicated?

This is a good example of how we crave for simplicity, but confuse it with superficiality. It seems that our lives have become so complicated, so busy, so hectic, that we do not want the additional complication of searching for the meaning of life. Superficiality then becomes a pseudo-simplicity and is expressed as the refusal to go to any psychological or spiritual depth. Traditional science and materialism feed into this. So then we are left with external complexity and internal superficiality. The Indian Yogi's way would be the opposite – external simplicity and internal depth. How can we shift our approach to life and ourselves towards how it should be?

My basic statement is that 'real bliss' is not possible in this material world of the senses (we shall try to define 'real bliss' later). We are all just chasing rainbows, and the rainbows surrounding us have multiplied and become more colourful, more powerful. We can't see the wood for the trees any more. We admire the colours and race after the pots of gold. 'It's here', 'No, it's the other end'. And while we chase from one end of the rainbow to the other, the rainbow moves and eventually disappears. We haven't found the pot of gold. Maybe if we had been quicker, more determined, found the rainbow sooner? We'll try again, go on 'rainbow watch', improve our stamina.

But what is behind rainbows? It is water and light and our senses. Our senses, eyes in this instance, perceive light (universal light, God's light) as rainbows when the light gets broken by water drops. Our sense of vision sees colours, and we follow our senses. And somebody, somewhere has told us that there is this pot of gold (bliss) if we're just quick enough.

We can apply this to all the other sensual things we chase. Take sex for example. Or even food. The same principle applies. It is the senses we follow.

Much of man's suffering in this world is caused by his inability to discrim-inate between good sensations and bad ones. ... [The] pleasant idea about a sensation causes an individual to repeat his experiences with that sensa-tion. When a sensation is constantly repeated, it causes a repetition of its corresponding pleasing idea. ... This mental habit – formed by repeating a pleasing idea that evolved from a sensation – is what causes the attractive-ness of sensations. Just as everybody is more or less in love with his own ideas about things, whether they are right or not, so also, the mind likes its own personal collection of mental sense habits. ... it is an idea that is liked by another idea.[30]

This is exactly what our consumerist culture uses – creating pleasant ideas and sense habits. Even further, the increasingly constant and immediate availability of pleasing ideas and objects does not even allow for a break during which we could question or slow down the course of events. And most of it happens at the level of ideas.

The objects of pleasing sense habits are increasingly always available. They might not be obtainable because of a shortage of money or other limitations. But even then, their potential availability can create much pain, longing, greed and envy. We are led to believe that bliss is just around the corner.

CHASING RAINBOWS (REFLECTION 2)

Sit or lie in a meditation position, close your eyes and consider the following questions for three minutes each. Just allow feelings, images, thoughts to come up in response to the questions. Don't expect a clear-cut answer. Reflect and explore.

1   *What ways of 'going inside' have you developed? Do you remember times when you used to do it quite naturally?*

2   *Do you know that 'little voice' inside you? What does it say? When do you hear it?*

3   *What is your pattern of acting against your 'better knowledge'? What are your habitual distractions?*

4   *What rainbows have you been chasing?*

Creativity and Fragmentation

This book is written by a psychotherapist; consequently there have been and will continue to be many mentions of psychotherapy. Psychotherapy and counselling seem to have become our Western way of 'going inside'. I think we need to move on now. Even though psychotherapy has been expressing the deep craving of our souls, I think it may be misleading us now. Different models are right at different times in the development of humanity. The great days of psychotherapy are over. James Hillman expresses it in the title of one of his books: *We've had one hundred years of psychotherapy and the world is getting worse.*

Where is psychotherapy going? Magazines are full of advertisements offering all kinds of self-development courses, personal growth experiences and alternative therapies, plus training, supervision, accreditation in all those approaches. This, no doubt, expresses a longing in our culture. The unconscious longing is for 'going inside', for re-connecting with Spirit.

Humanity today is suffering from spiritual malnutrition. People in parts of the world are suffering from physical starvation, but millions in all nations are suffering from spiritual starvation. Science has given the means to feed every person on this planet; it is man's spiritual poverty that makes him cling to selfishness and small-minded prejudices, thereby preventing him from eradicating hunger and other forms of deprivation.[31]

However, in psychotherapy as in most other areas of life, the ways and means to reach the goal have turned into goals in themselves. Even some forms of organised religion suffer from this means-goals-confusion, where for example going to church every Sunday has turned into the goal itself rather than being the means to reach God. As human beings we just have an intrinsic tendency to do that: The car, for example, used to be the means to get from A to B. Now, to have a sporty car, a big car, an expensive car, a four-wheel-drive car, have all turned into separate goals in their own right. We lose sight of the overall goal and become engrossed in sub-goals.

The world of gross matter, i.e. our world, is a world of fragmentation and splitting. We also have the ability to 'split' – an ability that has enabled us to create much of the complexity that surrounds us. And suddenly we cannot see the wood for the trees any more. Cars, for example, are now severely restricting the very purpose that they were initially built for – mobility. We experience immobility on the roads, immobility as a species. Pollution and global warming are suffocating us – physically and psychologically. We have the capacity to turn many things around like this, including psychotherapy and self-development. Our ability to analyse and to create complexity always seems to reach a point where the components or some of the characteristics of the components begin to work against us.

CREATIVITY

Our creativity seems to have an essential flaw, apart from the fact that it has become a goal in itself. It seems to be incapable of being 'just great'. Destructivity seems to be the travel companion of creativity, just as the universal forces of creation, preservation and dissolution operate together all around us. The more creative we become, the bigger the potential for destruction seems to grow. Creativity is trendy – the creative process, creative thinking, creative solutions, the creative manager, the internet. We are drowning in the outpourings of unlimited creativity. The advertising industry, more TV channels, more films, more games, faster information technology. We are creating more and faster, and no area of life is protected from our creativity tearing it to bits or blowing it up like a balloon. The creative process itself has become the object of our creative enquiry, and is being sold as a commodity.

Yet, we are creative beings living in a creative universe. To be alive is to create. Our creativity is not separate from the creativity of the universe. We are the result, and part of universal creation. However, unaware of the flip side of the coin, we have allowed our creativity and our capacity to fragment and split to form an unholy alliance. A lot of the human creative effort is driven by greed, envy, competition, profit. The arts and humanities in our schools, where children could learn and enjoy a deeper (and higher) and more responsible sense of creativity, have largely become side-issues. Even art itself has become primarily a commodity.

In his book *The Holographic Universe* Michael Talbot discusses the Jungian concept of synchronicity, coincidences that are so unusual and meaningful that they cannot be attributed to chance alone. Talbot writes:

> Peat [a physicist] believes that synchronicities are therefore 'flaws' in the fabric of reality, momentary fissures that allow us a brief glimpse of the immense and unitary order underlying all of nature. Put another way, Peat believes that synchronicities reveal the absence of division between the physical world and our inner psychological reality. Thus the relative scarcity of synchronous experiences in our lives shows not only the extent to which we have fragmented ourselves from the general field of consciousness, but also the degree to which we have sealed ourselves off from the infinite and dazzling potential of the deeper orders of mind and reality. According to Peat, when we experience a synchronicity, what we are really experiencing 'is the human mind operating, for a moment, in its true order and extending throughout society and nature, moving through orders of increasing subtlety, reaching past the source of mind and matter into creativity itself'.[32]

Compared to the above quote, the creativity that we have grown so used to, and that the advertising brainwashers are selling us feels flat. Only creativity beyond mind and matter can be without destruction. But we are trying to create the illusion of eternity and bliss (progress!) in the objects of our desires. So, we become convinced that

(1) we can create everything, just given time, and
(2) soul bliss can be found in objects (things, people, relationships, careers, money etc.).

Let us see how we are abusing our creativity in the vain attempt to create paradise on Earth, and thus heat up the hell we're living in.

PARADISE ON EARTH

I am driving along, at dusk, through a town. My car radio station has just turned to advertisements. It's all about buying more things, what to do with the things you've bought, and how to find out about yet more things to buy. Information technology is everywhere. Computer-created advertisements are grinning, shining, impressing on me from billboards. My head aches, I feel sick and over-loaded. I can't get away from it.

A parallel world created by human technology and science is surrounding us. It is a creation. God created the universe including us and he gave us the power to create as well. We like the idea of paradise, so we are trying to create it. But

God also created the apple tree. We too have the ability to create apple trees. That's where we got it wrong. We've put too much emphasis on the apple-trees. Temptation and teasing have become the motor of consumerism – a paradise of and for the senses. Our paradise has become an apple orchard, and we can't see the wood for the trees any more.

We are surrounded by objects – man-made objects. But then, as we are part of creation and thus of nature, our objects are also part of this world, universe, God. Just as evil is part of creation, we can create internal and external spaces for good and for evil. But could the fact that we have gone for the apples be a meaningful part of the whole story?

At one level, our consumerist, capitalist, rational, masculine approach to life has created people who are surrounded by a thick fog – the fog of objects and desires. The bright spark of spirit can hardly get through the fog. We're too busy finding our way in this fog to pay attention to the light that is trying to reach us.

But at another level there is meaning in it. Imagine the whole world immersed in a mist and the light can't get through. What is the challenge? Is it for the light to try harder, or for us to find ways of clearing the mist? Well, the light is trying harder. It is up to us to do our bit. But we don't know how to clear the mist. We are still trying to enjoy the promise that our creations hold – only the doubts as to whether we can ever reach 'the promised land' are getting a bit stronger.

And that's where the second part of the story comes in. We had to build the apple orchard, and create the fog so that we can use our second gift – free will. Creativity and free will are the two abilities that connect us to the universe. Brian Swimme sees human consciousness as the universe folding back on itself, and the universe becoming conscious of itself. Consciousness is not possible without creativity and free will. All three, consciousness, creativity and free will, are directly linked to the universe, to God. As energies they are trying to maintain the link with their cosmic source. They need to maintain the link with their cosmic source, because ultimately they are only a reflection of it, for otherwise they would not exist.

This is where I see our challenge. We are using so much consciousness, creativity and will-power in our futile attempts to create paradise on Earth, and we forget that those qualities are our soul-qualities, the reflections of spirit within us. The thick mist of objects, consumerism, greed and envy with which we have surrounded ourselves, disconnects us from God.

Consciousness has turned into the scientific rationality that sees the world and other people as 'things' to be exploited and explained. Creativity is abused for producing and selling more things, and for creating more needs. Willpower is used for competition and power over things and other people. But we have free will and we can choose. The drama around us and within is urging us to choose.

CREATIVITY (REFLECTION 3)

Sit or lie in a meditation position, close your eyes and consider the following questions for three minutes each. Just allow feelings, images, thoughts to come up in response to the questions. Don't expect a clear-cut answer. Reflect and explore.

1   *How open or closed are you to seeing and experiencing yourself as a soul-being? How far have you limited your consciousness to the scientific rationality that tries to know and explain everything by using our Western scientific models?*

2   *How much of your creativity is used in a purely commercial way and entirely related to 'managing your life'?*

3   *How much of your will-power has been reduced to having 'power over' things and people? How much do you equate will-power with control?*

Maps for the Inner Journey

It should be becoming clearer by now that our inner and the outer worlds are not that different, possibly much more similar than we think, and even 'made from the same stuff'. In the previous chapters there have been explicit and implicit hints at holistic and holographic thinking, which is quite the opposite of our normal way of splitting and fragmenting. We split something up into fragments which often cannot easily be split. Why are we doing that, and how can we stop doing it? The reasons why we should stop splitting should be clear by now – it is about our evolution as spiritual human beings and it has also become a matter of the survival of the human species.

There are different levels of splitting that we are engaged in – inner and outer, psychological and social, personal and interpersonal. We are surrounded by splitting processes and our inner world is filled with them as well. Remember, craving for certainty and addicted to conflict? There is a psychological level of splitting and fragmentation, which gets addressed and analysed by many psychological theories. There is also a psycho-social-spiritual level, which we will address further on using the psychological greenhouse. But underneath all these different levels is the fact that the world of matter is 'split off from spirit' and that the world of matter is governed by the law of splitting (or the law of duality). It is the process of ahamkara (see Chapter 2). In order to go beyond duality, we need to go inside. The only way out of this world of splitting is to go inside and beyond the world of matter, so why not ignore all the superficial levels and go to the deeper one right away? Why all those words? We want straight and simple answers: 'Just tell me what to do, and that's that then.'

If it was that easy, our planet would be crowded with enlightened people. That is obviously not the case. So it must be fairly difficult to get beyond duality. In order to fully take on board the very fundamental assertion that the only way out is in, we need to do something that is like slowly peeling back the layers of an onion. We need maps that guide us gradually to the core of intuitive under-standing. Going to that core too quickly can lead to much confusion and set-backs. Our accustomed way of seeing and thinking about things has grown over a long time. It needs time and effort to change the programming of our mind. Our governing blinkered and conditioned rational or outer mind, with all its ways of perceiving and thinking in the ways of splitting and duality, will not give up its conditioning so easily. This is particularly true if the old, habitual ways of seeing things are driven by unconscious and repressed motives, i.e. motives that were relevant in childhood, but are now still operating unconsciously. This is the case for most of us and, as we have explored earlier, it is this unconscious moti-vation that is being used, abused and strengthened by the culture of consumerism and materialism.

In the following chapters we shall develop maps and models for the rational mind that will help us change our habitual conditioned ways of seeing and expe-riencing ourselves and our world. I am using the term 'map' here because I am trying to take you on a journey into unknown territory. The territory is your own inner world; the destination is your soul. The journey has to go through the different levels of your mind, your consciousness and your intellect.

So far we have been addressing the rational mind in order to find a way through to the intuitive mind. The rational mind will need some convincing and some maps that make sense in order to allow this to happen. The maps will open the mind so it can let go of many of the blinkers towards spirituality that have been created in our heads. The maps are for the rational mind, because we need its co-operation on our quest.

Everybody who has tried to meditate knows how strong the 'blinkered' rational or outer mind, which is often described as a monkey, can be. As soon as you close your eyes, all sorts of thoughts and images start appearing – shopping lists, things that need to be done, memories, fantasies. The mind is attached to its old ways because those ways appear to be the total truth that has served us and helped us to survive so far. But have they really? What are those old ways about and where do they come from anyway?

Why then is the mind so afraid of being empty, the prerequisite for deep medi-tation? So afraid of being still, or allowing us to go to that place of stillness inside? Well, for the rational mind the world is 'as it is'. It sees things as they apparently are. The Eastern wisdom would say that our rational mind sees maya and is part of maya, the world of matter, the world of delusion. At this stage of drawing the maps, let us just agree that the rational mind is trained by our education, our history, and by our conventions – in short, it has lots of maps that are sort of 'matter of fact' ones. For that part of our mind, to be still and empty would mean something like death. That part of our mind sees, interprets and considers the world of matter, and the laws, rules and regulations that apply in this world.

Models are strange things. We rely on them so much. They help us see and then they can also blind us. But then, they are no more than symbols – like the written word. We think in symbols. Our symbols create and reflect our world. And then again, we can drown the soul in a world of symbols. Soul-connection means going beyond or behind the symbols. The following maps encourage you to go behind the symbols. You can do that by personalising the maps. Each map will contain Reflections which will help you with your personal journey inside.

5

Splitting and Boundaries

There we are, surrounded by the objects of our creativity, onto which we have projected our emotional needs and desires, our growth and often our whole life journey. Here is another claustrophobic car story.

I am sitting in my car, stuck in a huge traffic jam. It is one of those very hot and humid summer days that we have been getting lately. I am sweating. I'd love to open the car window, but I know that then I would breathe in the fumes of all those other cars around me even more directly. Even though there aren't any clouds around, the air looks misty, with a yellow-reddish glow. Aeroplanes are flying low over my head, carrying vast numbers of fellow humans to their destinations. The weather-forecast man on the radio says the air quality in London will be very poor today. My eyes feel sore and my nose is running; my head is thinking how to make up for my delay in getting to my destination: I'll be running late, again. I feel imprisoned – in my car, in between appointments, in the air around me that I have to breathe, in the heat, the deadlines, the destinations, the cars and people around me and above me. Even the car radio, producing the most human sounds around me, feels inhuman, an intrusion.

In this situation I am surrounded by a metal box, my feet are on a metal floor, the rubber tyres are in contact with the asphalt. I am not in contact with the earth. Above me, my contact with the sky is blocked by pollution, aeroplanes and noise. Even my most intimate interaction with my environment, through my breathing, is blocked by pollutants and by the smell of car exhaust fumes. And I am rushing between manmade objects, from A to B to C to D, disconnected from Earth and Heaven, disconnected from my inner Self.

I listen to the weather forecast on a London radio station on what must be one of the hottest days this year; words like 'glorious sunshine' and 'fine weather' flow freely. A mete-orologist is explaining the reasons for this sudden change from the coldest May in years to temperatures higher than in Nairobi and L.A. 'We now all agree that global warming as a result of pollution is happening,' he says. 'Does that mean we can all look forward to a gloriously hot summer?' asks the interviewer in response. Government smog alerts are issued (which, again, is meaningless because nobody knows what it means and what to do about it, apart from the fact that people with asthma need to be careful).

Some of my patients start their session off by commenting on the wonderful weather. Sometimes I cannot hold back and explain why I do not like the glorious sunshine. Then

they look disappointed, like children whose toys have just been spoiled. I want to scream:
'The planet is dying, and all you're worried about is your sun-tan.' But I don't scream.

But how dare the media treat us like children? Why do we allow them to treat us like toddlers? Sunshine is wonderful – the picture-book mentality of fifty years ago is poured into our brains. This is frequently followed directly by stories about pollution and global warming. Why do the news-people not make the connections? Do they not see it or do they not want to pass it on to us? The psychological part of the answer lies in the mechanism of 'splitting'.

As children we learn to split between good things and bad things. Mother is either completely good or completely bad. We are either completely good or completely bad. Growing up then means to learn about complexity. The same person or thing can be good and bad at different times or even at the same time. We can like *and* dislike; we can love *and* hate. However, many of us get stuck in the black or white seeing and thinking of 'splitting', especially when we grow up with parents or in a culture where splitting is very common and has become the main survival strategy.

Our culture, our world has become incredibly complex and incredibly fast. Increasingly we are only able to comprehend often disconnected and contradictory fragments of it. And more and more we are only fed fragments of information – sound bytes, visual bytes, feeling bytes. We are enticed to use our deeply ingrained infantile capacity for splitting to maintain a sense of security and simplicity in an increasingly complex world.

To connect glorious sunshine with the frightening and largely unpredictable threat of global warming is complicated and might give us a headache. As long as we separate the two we can enjoy the warmth of the sun, and see pollution and climatic changes as an abstract and far-away issue.

Ecologists say that we need to change our attitudes and see the whole rather than separate fragments if we want to stop or slow down the decline of the planet. The changes and challenges are big, really big. In a few decades southern England is predicted to have harsh, burning and pitiless summers, and bitterly cold winters. The north may turn into a wine growing Mediterranean region – quite pleasant. Brighton and other seaside towns could be swallowed up by the rising sea levels from the melting polar caps.

This may sound like science fiction, but there are too many experts now who are sure that the process is well on its way. The most worrying aspect of the whole scenario is that the climatic changes are unpredictable. We do not know what will happen. We are facing a global uncertainty that will leave none of us untouched. The climatic crisis, and not just the widespread ignorance about it, is directly related to our ability to split and fragment – industrialisation and exploitation of our planet's resources for often greedy purposes without taking the whole picture into account, without going to our inner wisdom (soul) first and trying to see from that perspective. The succession of crises that rumble through the global financial markets is very similar. There we have split off money from its original purpose of simplifying the exchange of goods and have created a bloated and largely artificial market for money itself. Again, through splitting and fragmentation without the necessary holistic considerations we have created monsters that are turning against us. It is this partial and fragmented discovery and application of universal laws without a soul-perspective that is causing many of the crises we are facing – like BSE, like wars, like pollution, like many illnesses.

How can we cope with the consequences of our *blind actions*, which affect all of us so acutely? Are we ready for slowing down and possibly reversing the processes that have already started, and for living with the consequences of those conditions that we cannot change? These questions cannot be answered easily, but we will surely be badly prepared if we continue to split our world and ourselves apart, instead of acquiring a deep inner attitude that sees the multitude of connections in and between our inner and outer worlds. And this is where all the information-producers and feeders, like teachers, media people, politicians, even psychotherapists, ought to feel a growing responsibility. We need to get away from feeding people disconnected bits of the world just for the sake of blasting more bits and bytes through the wires and the ether. We have the opportunity to help people see the inter-connectedness of everything, so that we have a chance to feel part of the global interdependent community that we really are. From that point we can reach out to the universe. Quality instead of quantity of information is needed in all areas of our lives.

Boundaries

Our capacity to split is so deeply ingrained that it feels almost impossible to develop a more holistic approach to ourselves and to life. This is because the mechanisms of splitting, rooted in the duality of the world of matter and in the ego (ahamkara), permeate our psyche and our consciousness to such an extent that they represent *reality* for us. These processes create our outer mind, and it is the interaction between outer mind and outer world that creates our apparent reality. We shall now move on and explore the internal origins and psychological dynamics of splitting and fragmentation that we all carry inside. We need to understand them before we can overcome them.

One of Ken Wilber's first books was entitled *No Boundary*. Since then he has written and published many others in his usual brilliant style, analysing our world from a mainly Buddhist philosophical perspective. *No Boundary* is special though, because in it he deals in a simple and straightforward way with the issues of splitting and fragmentation. In good Eastern tradition he argues that all our boundaries are our own creation and that they do not really exist. On our journey inside to the point where we can begin to experience that state of one-ness, of no separation, no splitting, we need to get our head round the issue of boundaries, because they are so real, so energy draining and ultimately so limiting and even destructive. We need to understand where the boundaries come from if we want to transcend them. This is an important layer of the onion.

In the Sankhya system splitting and fragmentation are a function of ahamkara, the ego. This is seen as a state which needs to be transcended for healing and self-development to occur. Western psychology and psychotherapy have developed many complex and fascinating models and theories about psychological splitting. These theories can throw light on many of the psychological disorders that can arise when the splitting (separation) process goes wrong, but they do not really show us a way out of and beyond it (meaning beyond the ego). Western psychological models are usually limited to 'normal ego development'.

We shall now use some of those Western models as maps to understand the intricacies of the ego and of the sense-mind. But we are not aiming at finding a 'benign' form of splitting and fragmentation or a 'healthy' ego-structure as Western psychology would attempt. Although such a process of developing a better ego-structure may be necessary for some people, our premise here is that our consciousness needs to transcend the ego if we want to get to soul.

OBJECT RELATIONS THEORY

Psychoanalytic 'object relations theory' ('object' here means 'the object of the internal experience') deals with the issues and psychological problems that can arise in the process of a human infant separating and individuating from mother, which ultimately is the process of setting boundaries between 'self' and 'other'. Initially, it is assumed, the infant has no concept of himself being separate from its environment. The process of setting the first boundaries is seen as necessary for the development of a self-image and as essential for survival.

The infant needs to learn to differentiate between 'self' and 'other', good and bad, pleasure and pain. However, many things can go wrong in this process. For example, if the child is faced with a cold and rejecting mother, it needs to reconcile this in its psyche by splitting off its terror, anger and pain, because those feelings about the primary care-taker cannot be expressed, as they might threaten the child's own survival, which is dependent on being cared for. A positive, caring image of mother is being maintained at all cost.

There are various forms of inappropriate intra-psychic 'splitting' that can take place in this process of 'keeping mother good even when she isn't'. Object relations theory ultimately sees this as the condition that can lead to narcissistic, schizoid or borderline personality disorders. Without going into more detail of the theory, it is easy to comprehend how this first separation and self-image and other-image building process of the infant can set the scene for all future ones. The disorders of the self are then seen as the failure to develop a stable, cohesive, separate and individuated self. Typical splitting attitudes would be: I am good, you are bad; I am bad, you are good. These patterns are seen as a result of the infant's 'separation-individuation process' having been arrested (not completed), usually between the ages of one and three. As a result borderline and narcissistic personality disorders can develop.

In the borderline personality, the self and the object, which is the internal representation of mother, are both split between 'good' and 'bad' and 'object constancy' is not developed, because the object, i.e. internal representation of mother, constantly fluctuates between good and bad. Object constancy refers to the ability of the child to 'hold' in his psyche a constant picture of mother in her conflicting aspects, which were up to then experienced as separate ones: good and bad, love and hate, present and absent.

In the narcissistic personality the developmental arrest is also assumed to happen during the individuation-separation phase. The self does not achieve a mature separation from mother and therefore develops difficulties in sharing, empathy, and in acknowledging the thoughts, feelings and needs of others. These failures are often concealed and latent and become manifest later in life during periods of disappointment or trauma when narcissistic supply lines dry up or fail.

As a result of these impairments a 'false defensive self' is assumed to develop, which relates to the real world through a maladaptive ego structure. The patient experiences this as a sense of discontinuity, fragility, or unstable self-identity, and as confusions between fantasies of what she contains and what people are like with the reality of what she contains and what people are really like. All these impairments are seen as a consequence of the underlying 'abandonment depression' against which the patient feels she must defend at all costs.

Essentially the model describes the origin of people's confused boundaries. As a result of those confused boundaries they cannot come into relationship with themselves or with others; they see themselves in others and others in themselves; they love others when they want to love themselves; they hate themselves when they want to hate their parents. It is easy to see how such a confusion between self and others can lead to problems in the relationships a person has with parts of herself and with other people.

Psychotherapy would then aim at addressing and strengthening the patient's 'real self' through a range of therapeutic means. One of the most skilful therapeutic methods is the 'art of confrontation' with the borderline patient. What is confronted in an empathic, introspective, and creative way is the borderline patient's (her false self's) sole aim in therapy, which is primarily to 'feel better' at all cost. In order to achieve this, the patient either tries to turn the therapist into a 'primary caretaker', or into someone onto whom she can project her painful feelings. The therapist is made either 'all good' or 'all bad', according to the internal splitting dynamic. In therapy sessions these strategies of the patient's false self are confronted in order to continuously address and strengthen the glimpses of 'real self' that might be there. This often leads to the patient having to face the underlying abandonment depression, which is the point in therapy when proper individuation and separation can take place, thus leading to the patient developing a 'mature and fused self'.

As complex as the theory may look, I think in practice all therapists have faced patients' projections, their 'acting out' behaviours, and have struggled to maintain boundaries in order to contain the chaos. The assumption that there is a 'real self' somewhere, which is being served by our struggles, is not only a nice motivator, but this 'real self' actually becomes visible in the therapy room. The frustration in this phase of therapy is when I, as the therapist, can see the glimpses of 'real self' in the patient, but the patient cannot. Usually there is no point in just telling the patient what I see, because the 'false self' will fiercely defend against any such insights, as they entail the danger of having to face the abandonment depression.

Object relations theory deals with the psychological disorders that can be caused as a result of a wrong and defensive setting of the very first boundaries between self and others, and between good and bad. This development is fuelled by the fear of annihilation, i.e. the abandonment depression. The therapeutic relationship then becomes the main healing factor in therapy and serves as a microcosm where the old boundaries are destroyed and more appropriate internal and external ones are built. In order to withstand the bombardment of projections, transference and counter-transference, the therapist himself needs to set clear boundaries for the therapeutic encounter.

How does this then fit with our notion that all boundaries between ourselves and others and between different parts of our own inner selves are ultimately an illusion in the face of the one-ness of everything? How can we invest a lot of time and energy into helping people to establish 'proper' boundaries if ultimately boundaries are an illusion, and the one-ness of all is the ultimate reality? Could the assumed failure to establish object constancy be a reflection of the fact that such constancy is essentially not possible in the world of duality? Could personality disorders be seen as just an extreme experience of the duality and contradictions of matter?

To some extent object relations theory confirms that boundaries are an illusion, that they relate to the self-image which is all 'in the mind'. It is obviously not given from birth, but rather something that develops in the infant's psyche (the mind) in the very first stages of life; and the development of that mental construct is the result of complex psychological (mental) processes. So object relations theory would probably agree with the spiritual teachings that say that the sense of the separate self is an 'illusion' or a mental construct. But object relations theory does not have a spiritual perspective. It does not deal with the polarity of 'boundaries vs. no boundaries', but concentrates on 'pathological boundaries vs. appropriate boundaries'.

As with all models, the object relations model covers one aspect and one level of reality. It explains the struggle of the human infant to develop boundaries and to become an individual. It also explains very well the psychological damage that can happen, and that can dominate the adult's life later on. It makes sense that therapies based on this model will focus on repairing the damage that was incurred in the process. The aim in therapy will be the building of appropriate boundaries, i.e. the development of an ego structure that can function relatively smoothly in the world without being constantly torn between opposites of good and bad, love and hate in the relationship with oneself and with others. However, from a spiritual angle we also need to note that this therapeutic 'repair job' may well create the illusion that a life without contradictions and conflict can be possible.

We need a wider context, one that includes both the setting and the elimination of boundaries, if we want to understand how we can get to the state of union that we want to achieve by going inside. Otherwise the 'setting of boundaries' can turn into an excessive 'boundary making', which creates people who are very well protected, have clear boundaries, but have somehow lost spontaneity, joy and trust in the process.

There is another possible dilemma in the object relations model, if we take it as the total truth. Perhaps, the boundary confusion that the model considers pathological, i.e. in the narcissistic and borderline personalities, is a call from the soul for the elimination of boundaries. Perhaps the pathology is just the way in which the ego misunderstands a deeper soul-call.

This leaves us with a dilemma that we are going to encounter with all the psychological models that we shall be using as maps on our journey. As long as the theories behind the models do not explicitly include a spiritual perspective, they have the potential to lead to confusion between ego and soul. We could compare the situation of the psychotherapy of 'personality disorders' with the treatment of cancer. For example, even when we know that a certain cancer is clearly environmental in origin, we would still want to treat the person who is suffering the cancer as best we can and even with treatment methods that may not include the environmental perspective at all. The same applies to psychotherapy even when it does not have a soul perspective. However, proper healing always takes place at a soul level, which may or may not include direct attempts at repairing body and mind.

THE BIRTH PROCESS AND BOUNDARIES

The Chill

When the fear comes,
Creeping in through some back-doors,
That have never been properly shut.

I go and look for the doors,
But fear has already surrounded me with a cold chill.
It's difficult to search in the dark,
While my body shivers and trembles.

I can sense the open doors – somewhere there,
Deep in the dark,
From where the draughty chill comes.

This is not the warm soothing darkness,
That I expected in the womb.

And then I know,
That the chill is coming from my mother's heart.

Grof's model of *basic perinatal matrices* (BPMs) is one of the most influential models in transpersonal psychology, and I think that it can help us to expand the boundary map. Grof is an American psychiatrist who started his research into altered states of consciousness in the 1960s in Prague. Back then he used LSD, nowadays he uses a breathing technique called *holotropic breathwork* to induce altered states. In his recent book *The Cosmic Game*[33] Grof gives a comprehensive account of his and his patients' learning from going inside in this particular way. Grof found that in altered states of consciousness people have transpersonal, cosmic unity, and birth experiences. From his observations he concludes that certain emotional life patterns have their origin in the birth process. While psycho-analytical models would look back no further than the first year of life, here we have a model that looks at the very initial process of boundary setting that a human being goes through in this life – the perinatal process.

On the basis of his research with altered states of consciousness, Grof defines the specific biological, psychological, archetypal and spiritual aspects of each of the four BPMs.

Perinatal phenomena occur in four distinct experiential patterns, which I call the Basic Perinatal Matrices (BPMs). Each of these four matrices is closely related to one of the four consecutive periods of biological delivery. At each of these stages, the baby undergoes experiences that are character-ized by specific emotions and physical feelings; each of these stages also seems to be associated with specific symbolic images. These come to repre-sent highly individualized psychospiritual blueprints that guide the way we experience our lives. They may be reflected in individual and social psychopathology, or in religion, art, philosophy, politics, and other areas of life. And, of course, we gain access to these psychospiritual blueprints through non-ordinary states of consciousness, which allow us to see the guiding forces of our lives much more clearly.[34]

Understandably, Grof's way of connecting birth, biological, and spiritual elements in his model has made it attractive to transpersonal psychotherapies like psychosynthesis. Within psychosynthesis the model has been applied to key concepts like subpersonalities, the qualities of will and love, and mind-sets. We shall ponder the model here in its relevance to the question of boundaries.

TABLE 1: PSYCHO-SPIRITUAL COMPONENTS OF THE BPMs

	BPM 1	BPM 2	BPM 3	BPM 4
Psychospiritual symbolism	Amniotic universe	Cosmic engulfment	Death and rebirth struggle	Death and rebirth
Physical process	In womb prior to delivery.	Contractions begin, but cervix closed.	Moving through birth canal.	Leaving mother's body.
Psychological experience	Symbiotic union with mother, timelessness, in touch with infinity.	Antagonism with mother, experience of 'no exit', hopelessness, mistrust, loneliness, never-ending suffering.	Light at the end of the tunnel, intensification of suffering and tension, ecstasy with aggressive and destructive elements.	Separation from mother, forming a new relationship with her, death-rebirth experience, ego-death.
Potential Psycho-pathology	Mystic subpersonality, selfishness, conflict avoidance, sense of impotence.	Victim subpersonality, desire for unity & self-doubt, no choice - environment is causal.	Rebel and crusader subpersonality, fiercely independent, blaming.	Doubting, fearful subpersonality, longing to be back in BPM 1, unsettled, no home, lonely.
Task in life	To enter into the world and its struggles.	Learn to accept pain, separation and dependence.	Move on to co-operation, forgiveness and compassion.	Realise the potential of selflessness, brotherhood and unconditional love.

Obviously, the process of birth is the one in which new-born child is for the very first time faced with the need to establish her separateness from mother, i.e. her boundaries as an individual. This process of individuation and separation then continues over the years of growing up.

Table 1 lists the different BPM stages and their psycho-spiritual components. It shows that the model is one of differentiation and separation (BPM 1 to BPM 3), finally leading to a new stage of relationship (BPM 4).

In his research Grof found that these four stages recur as themes and key issues throughout people's lives. He sees these stages as setting up COEX (Constellations of Condensed Experience) systems in people's unconscious, which act as dynamic governing systems that have a function at a specific level of the unconscious.

Each COEX has a theme that characterizes it. For example, a single COEX constellation can contain all major memories of events that were humiliating, degrading, or shameful. The common denominator of another

COEX might be the terror of experiences that involved claustrophobia, suffocation, and feelings associated with oppressing and confining circumstances. Rejection and emotional deprivation leading to our distrust of other people is another very common COEX motif. ... Each COEX constellation seems to be superimposed over and anchored into a very particular aspect of the birth experience.[35]

But COEX systems can have even deeper roots, according to Grof. The material he has collected from his clients over the years also seems to contain images and experiences that relate to past lives, archetypes of the 'collective unconscious', and even identification with other life forms and universal processes like creation and dissolution of galaxies and even universes. In his conclusions Grof assigns a spiritual quality to his proposed COEX system. He feels that they form the basic patterns that mediate between an individual and the universe: external events can activate corresponding COEX systems; COEX systems shape our perception, and then we act to bring about situations in reality that echo our COEX patterns. According to this model we are constantly re-creating inner psychological patterns in the external world.

Obviously, from the point of view of the establishment of boundaries, BPM 4 is the most interesting pattern because it is the final separation from the womb, from mother, and the emergence from the dark struggles of BPM 3. Grof calls it the 'death and rebirth experience', which has a distinct symbolic and spiritual dimension. In their altered states his subjects often relived this phase as a death-rebirth experience. Grof interprets this as 'ego-death', where the false ego gets eliminated at all levels, emotional, intellectual and spiritual, and a more realistic image of the world can be developed.

According to Grof this 'hitting rock bottom' experience can then lead on to higher spiritual experiences like merging with the rest of the world, and the appreciation of natural beauty and simplicity.

Grof goes on to describe the transpersonal potential in the experience of the BPM 4 matrix:

Higher motivating forces, such as the pursuit of justice, the appreciation for harmony and beauty and the desire to create it, a new tolerance and respect for others, as well as feelings of love, become increasingly important in our lives. What is more, we perceive these as direct, natural, and logical expressions of our true nature and of the universal order.[36]

Here we have a metaphor for the way in which separation and annihilation can lead to a new stage of inter-dependence and one-ness. It seems somewhat similar to the way in which in so-called 'personality disorders' the abandonment depression needs to be faced and worked through before the 'real self' can emerge. In terms of boundaries it seems to imply that the complete formation of boundaries is necessary before all boundaries can be eliminated.

The BPM model, as a COEX, is assumed to also apply to other stages of human development, i.e. childhood (BPM 1), adolescence (BPM 2), adulthood (BPM 3), mid-life crisis (BPM 4). We may even be able to see the development of humanity through the eyes of this model. We could see that humanity has been stuck in BPM 3 for a long time and is even reaching something like ego-death, where previous certainties are being replaced by large-scale uncertainties on many levels. But at the same time glimpses of BPM 4 are emerging as selflessness, brotherhood and unconditional love in many political, ecological and spiritual movements.

The object relations model of boundaries (see above) seems to address issues that arise in the development from BPM 1 to BPM 3. The borderline personality disorder could be said to represent stuckness between BPM 2 and BPM 3. Here the separation process never moves on to the potential interdependence of BPM 4, but oscillates between dependence and independence, antagonism and synergism, victim and rebel, self-doubt and blame. The narcissistic personality disorder represents a similar arrest, but it includes the energies of BPM 1 in its manifestation. We might even say that here BPM 1 and BPM 4 get confused, and the turbulence of 2 and 3 are avoided by retreating back into BPM 1, back into the positive womb. This narcissistic pattern of retreating back into the BPM 1 state can often be seen in people who follow certain pseudo-spiritual paths, and who use their so-called spirituality to avoid the struggles of everyday life. As I shall argue later, any spiritual path that does not have a clear concept of devotion is in danger of being abused for the BPM 1 pattern of narcissistic ego-inflation.

In both the borderline and the narcissistic patterns, it is the terror of the abandonment depression that leads to the failure of the development of appropriate boundaries, and thus to the failure of achieving the synthesis state of BPM 4, where boundaries can be dissolved within a higher context.

The implications of both models for ego-centred psychotherapy are fairly clear. Psychoanalytical approaches probably guide people out of the stuckness of the first three BPMs by helping the establishment of proper boundaries, thus leading to independence. However, they are unlikely to facilitate the further step into BPM 4, which is the step towards inter-dependence, and ultimately towards the elimination of boundaries. Many political events around us can be seen in similar terms. For example, the process of German unification involved the sudden elimination of boundaries, not in order to move towards BPM 4 type inter-dependence, but rather in order to move back to some kind of 'primal union' (BPM 1). The step the other way would have involved the letting go of the 'egos' of the two Germanys and facing the underlying abandonment depression, in this case the still unresolved and repressed reasons that led to the division in the first place. As a result the separation and conflicts between East and West- Germany are still very strong ten years on. The pathologies of BPM 2 and 3 are still being acted out, especially in the east where there are many incidents of right-wing violence against foreigners.

The main conclusion that we can draw from the model of boundaries and BPMs is: no gain without pain. In order to get to BPM 4 we need to have left 1, 2 and 3 behind, certainly as much as they can be left behind. Otherwise, what might appear as a spiritual path could be a running back into the safety and security of BPM 1 (the womb). This corresponds well with the messages that we receive from the religions of the world. Enlightenment is not easy. It requires discipline, hard work; and trials must be faced with courage and determination.

LIMITATIONS OF THE MODELS

The two models, object relations theory and the BPMs, analyse and clarify how splitting and fragmentation develop as dynamic forces in our psyche. We can easily see how certain patterns can solidify and how people can then struggle with the same issues again and again. Psychotherapy can help them out of the stuckness by helping them to:-

a) face the feared depression that the pattern is meant to defend against and realising that the fear belongs to childhood survival fears, and to

b) establish appropriate boundaries and developing the will and courage to move on, possibly towards BPM 4.

The object relations model clearly has no spiritual perspective, while the BPM model does. But I think we need to be careful and not confuse the BPM-model and the associated technique of holotropic breathwork with a spiritual path. As we shall see later, similar words of caution apply to psychosynthesis psychotherapy.

I think the problem with Grof's model is that he does not differentiate between subconscious and superconscious material. For him there does not seem to be a qualitative difference between, say, the experience of God in an altered state of consciousness or the experience of the claustrophobia of BPM 2. However, in Yogananda's teaching and in Vedic psychology the first would belong to the superconscious (or the soul) whereas the latter would belong to the subconscious (or the ego). This differentiation is important as we shall understand later.

We can appreciate how Grof's model deepens our understanding of the splitting dynamics that operate in our world of duality. The BPMs show us how the energies of conflict, struggle, separation, letting go of unity and of trying to relate to the source of unity from a position of separation are represented and come alive in the birth process. But we must not forget that it is a universal law that is being acted out here. The same laws probably apply to the formation of galaxies as well as the birth of human beings.

The process that Grof describes with the BPMs starts at a point when the soul is already incarnated, which happens at the point of conception. Going back to that process in an altered state of consciousness means going back to the very first phases of the soul's incarnation. Hence, pre-incarnation memories from the superconscious, from previous lives, from states of being united with spirit, are likely to be still more present than later on when a lot of mental memory space is occupied with experiences from this life. But the unity in the womb already is a separation from spirit. It is qualitatively different from pre-incarnation experiences.

It is like the Big Bang, the now widely agreed starting point of our universe. We can go back to the very first milliseconds of the birth of the universe. But this does not tell us anything about what was there before the Big Bang. It does not answer the *Why* question. This is exactly the point where I think Grof may have got it wrong. He has discovered a pattern of the world of matter in human life, a pattern that goes back to the very beginnings and can therefore additionally give glimpses of what was there before. But what was there before is qualitatively different, because it comes from a different (transcendental) dimension, and needs to be treated as such. Therefore, the material that gets evoked in the transpersonal experiences through holotropic breathwork needs to be carefully analysed as belonging either to the incarnate realm (subconscious) or to the pre-incarnate realm (superconscious). This is very important, because, as we shall see later, the spiritual path is about connecting with the superconscious while letting go of the subconscious.

The parallel in cosmology would be that scientists with their observations and calculations have gone all the way back to the Big Bang, and are now discovering that the dynamics of matter, which had been the focus of their inquiries, seem to be much less causal than the vacuum (the void, nothingness). This qualitative shift, which is happening in cosmology, is missing in Grof's explorations.

No Boundary

We can now return to Ken Wilber's 'no boundary' model. The BPM model implies that the move towards no boundaries has to go through the stages of individuation and separation with the establishment of proper boundaries. Both object relations and BPM models show how we can get stuck in this development, and how an illusory or premature move towards no boundaries can be nothing more than a regressive move back into the 'positive womb' (BPM 1). In order to get to inter-dependence, to partnership with ourselves and between ourselves and others and our environment, we need to go through the 'mined field'; we need to go through the fears and the separations, the depressions and the loneliness. However, this critique of the models also indicates that a more direct path towards spiritual unity might be possible, thus avoiding the drama of BPMs 2 and 3 as necessary steps.

We can now appreciate Ken Wilber's passionate pleas for the elimination of the boundaries that we have created in our consciousness. The following quotation seems to describe the development of rigid boundaries, characteristic of BPM 3:

The simple fact is that we live in a world of conflict and opposites because we live in a world of boundaries. Since every boundary line is also a battle line, here is the human predicament: the firmer one's boundaries, the more entrenched are one's battles. The more I hold on to pleasure, the more I necessarily fear pain. The more I pursue goodness, the more I am obsessed with evil. The more I seek success, the more I must dread failure. The harder I cling to life, the more terrifying death becomes. The more I value anything, the more obsessed I become with its loss. Most of our problems, in other words, are problems of boundaries and the opposites they create. Now our habitual way of trying to solve these problems is to attempt to eradicate one of the opposites. We handle the problem of good vs. evil by trying to exterminate evil. We handle the problem of life vs. death by trying to hide death under symbolic immortalities. In philosophy we handle conceptual opposites by dismissing one of the poles or trying to reduce it to the other. The materialist tries to reduce mind to matter, while the idealist tries to reduce matter to mind. The monists try to reduce plurality to unity, the pluralists try to explain unity as plurality.[37]

The striving for unity (certainty, perfection) is a deep craving that we have. But we have struggled so hard to establish our ego boundaries (BPM 1 to BPM 3), that we have come to regard all boundaries as real, and unification is only imaginable as the elimination of one side against the other. Rather than fighting for the elimination of boundaries, we fight for the elimination of the other side. It is a 'winning over' rather than a 'winning with'. The boundary is experienced as a battle line rather than a meeting point, because we had to battle so hard to establish our own first boundaries. As a result, the 'winning over' strategy dominates our society. Progress is defined as progress towards the positive, away from the negative. But there is not much evidence that, even after centuries of such attempted progress, humanity is any happier, any more content or at peace with itself. The opposite seems to be the case – there is more anxiety, frustration, alienation, meaninglessness, boredom in the midst of wealth and plenty.

It seems that 'progress' and unhappiness might well be flip sides of the same restless coin. For the very urge to 'progress' implies a discontent with the 'present' state of affairs, so that the more I seek progress the more acutely I feel discontent. In blindly pursuing progress, our civilisation has, in effect, institutionalised frustration. For in seeking to accentuate the positive and eliminate the negative, we have forgotten entirely that the positive is defined only in terms of the negative.[38]

Could it then be that the survival struggle for boundaries in the birth process is shaping even the scientific and philosophical approaches of our culture? Vedic philosophy would place the origins of the boundary issue even deeper, at the very core of our existence – the world of matter is not even imaginable without duality, without opposites, without boundaries. Think about it: light requires dark, hot requires cold to be understood, to be experienced. Even my writing is part of the same pattern: words and no words, beginning and end.

But our culture seems to have pushed the boundary model to the extreme. It has created 'boundary realities' beyond the birth experience and beyond the basic characteristics of matter, in language, politics, societal structures, production and consumption, economics, science, and philosophy. All those realities have their own separating dynamics and make up the world into which we are born. They form the context which we enter through our birth struggle. We enter a 'BPM 3 world', full of rigid boundaries. It is not surprising that we get stuck at the same level and thus contribute to the stuckness of our culture. It is this realisation of the connectedness between inner and outer conditions that leads us to the under-standing that inner (psychological) and outer (societal) changes cannot be separated, and that the work on one level requires work on the other as well. The danger of having yet another boundary, namely the one between 'inner' and 'outer', is a particular pitfall for psychotherapy.

This separation between inner and outer is altogether an illusion, Wilber argues:

> We all have the feeling of 'self' on the one hand and the feeling of the external world on the other. But if we carefully look at the sensation of 'self-in-here' and the sensation of 'world-out-there', we will find that these two are actually one and the same feeling. In other words, what I now feel to be the objective world out there is the same thing I feel to be the subjective self in here. The split between the experiencer and the world of experiences does not exist, and therefore cannot be found...
> Surely, there aren't three separate entities here. Is there ever such a thing as a seer without seeing or without something seen? Is there ever seeing without a seer or without something seen? The fact is, the seer, seeing and the seen are all aspects of one process – never at any time is one of them found without the others.[39]

Sometimes we all experience our selves and our experience as a unity, without boundaries. This can be as a 'peak experience', as sexual orgasm, or when we need to be right here 'in the moment' with our whole being, like when we play tennis or squash, or when we ride a bicycle up a steep hill. However, we want to have this experience of unity not just as an occasional chance event or as a retro-grade escape from reality. We want to work towards re-discovering this sense of wholeness and connectedness as a permanent part of ourselves, because it is there and it belongs to us. And then we want to consciously approach reality from this sense of unity, and get involved in this BPM 3 world from a no-boundary soul-position. This is what 'the only way out is in' is all about – going inside to a place where boundaries do not exist, a place where we are connected with God and spirit. It is the place where we were right in the beginning (in BPM 1), before the process of ahamkara created the self-image in our minds.

Before we can develop a clearer map of the path that will lead us beyond boundaries, we need to explore further how entrenched the situation is. Entrenched, because the inner dynamics of boundary formation are completely linked with external dynamics, and that is why it all appears so real.

BOUNDARY ISSUES AND FEAR (REFLECTION 4)

Before moving on, I suggest that you spend a few moments considering your own boundary issues. Look at the list of issues in the left column of Table 2 and consider how each one operates in your life. Pay attention to the ones that ring bells. They are the issues that will keep you hooked on people, objects, or even alcohol, drugs. Having explored object relations theory and the BPM model in this chapter, you may even be able to connect some of the issues to the models. For example, 'I am terrified of rejection' is likely to be a BPM 2 issue, and chances are that rejection was used as a punishment in the infant's upbringing. 'I need to be in control' is more likely to be a BPM 3 issue, and it would hint at the infant's deep fear and insecurity about being loved with his weaknesses and vulnerabilities.

Looking at Table 2, do not forget that we all have boundary problems, because we are living in a world with boundary problems, and with an ego whose main task is the creation of boundaries, and all the splitting and fragmentation that this involves.

Now I would like you to consider two points in relation to those of the issues in column 1 that are particularly relevant to you:

1   *All those issues are created and maintained by fear. The second column lists some of the possible fear issues that can be connected with the boundary issues. You may also want to look back at Reflection 1 on page 30 and read the poem again. Ask yourself: What am I afraid of? Identify, as much as you can at this stage, where your personal fear comes from, and use column three for some notes on this.*

2   *Fear is 'the big issue'. In our fragmented world of duality a lot is run by fear – fear as a motivator, fear to sell goods and services, fear as protection, fear as control, fear as punishment. If you want to be on a spiritual path – as you most likely do because otherwise you would not be reading this – fear becomes an even bigger issue. The 'Bhagavad Gita' lists 26 ennobling soul-qualities that are important on the spiritual path and 'fearlessness' is the first one on the list. Yogananda writes in his commentary on the sacred Indian text:*

> *'Fearlessness (abhayam) is mentioned first because it is the impregnable rock on which the house of spiritual life must be erected. ... Fear robs man of the indomitability of his soul. Disrupting Nature's harmonious workings emanating from the source of divine power within, fear causes physical, mental, and spiritual disturbances. ... Fear ties the mind and heart (feeling) to the external man, causing the consciousness to be identified with mental or*

TABLE 2: BOUNDARIES AND FEAR

Boundary issue	Underlying fear issues	Add your own observations
I am a perfectionist.	Makes me feel safe. Outer order contains my inner chaos. Fear of failing.	
I can't be vulnerable.	Nobody will comfort me. There is no-one for me.	
I am terrified of rejection.	Expecting rejection.	
I have difficulties in forming or maintaining close relationships.	Fear of closeness, intimacy. Don't know what closeness and intimacy are.	
I can't stand physical closeness.	Fear of being rejected. Shame.	
I put others' needs first.	Fear of not appearing 'good'. Fear of appearing selfish.	
I feel guilty when criticised.	Criticism is an attack. I am terrified of my anger.	
I need to be in control.	Only when I am in control do I feel safe.	
I am terrified of responsibility.	Fear of making mistakes.	
I feel a 'black hole' inside.	No firm self-image. Fear of love - can't trust it.	
I feel anxious or panicky for no reason.	Deep fear.	
I cannot identify my feelings.	Feelings are destructive and dangerous.	
I assume responsibility for how others feel.	I am bad and I fear that my badness can damage others.	

physical nervousness, thus keeping the soul concentrated on the ego, the body, and the objects of fear. The devotee should discard all misgivings, realizing them to be stumbling blocks that hinder his concentration on the imperturbable peace of the soul.'

Can we really safely say that, what is hidden behind all those complex psychological models that we have explored in this chapter is nothing more, nothing less than fear? Are we oversimplifying here, or are we getting to the core?

I think it is fear that lies behind all the other 'disordered' emotional states like anger, depression, addictions, even if it is ultimately the fear of death. Some psychologists would say that underneath fear there is always pain. I would say that fear is the fear of pain. It seems that the process of splitting (ahamkara) sets free that energy of fear. Psychotherapy can help, and is sometimes absolutely necessary, to reduce the fear through the transformation of some boundaries into more appropriate ones. But this book is about a more basic, transcendental approach to the problems of splitting and fear. Yogananda summarises such an approach:

> When subconscious fears repeatedly invade the mind, in spite of one's strong mental resistance, it is an indication of some deep-seated karmic pattern. The devotee must strive even harder to divert his attention by infusion of his conscious mind with thoughts of courage. Further, and most important, he should confide himself completely into God's trustworthy hands. To be fit for Self-realization, man must be fearless.[40]

You may notice that the above approach to fear is quite different from how psychotherapy would approach it. The origin is seen in karmic patterns, i.e. the effects of actions carried out in this or in previous lives. And whereas most psychotherapies would advocate 'working through' the fear, here the emphasis is on consciously inviting thoughts of courage, and confiding in God (a higher authority). The infusion of the conscious mind with thoughts of courage sounds very much like the approach that would be taken by cognitive therapy, where dysfunctional thinking patterns are counteracted and replaced by more beneficial thinking patterns. At this stage, I would like to say that the 'psychotherapeutic working through' is probably necessary for many people. However, the cautions I have expressed earlier apply, especially the danger of becoming engaged in a very long process of travelling the realms of the subconscious without ever reaching the superconscious. In particular those people who feel they are drawn to a spiritual path, (for example, even expressing an interest by reading this book) should try to include the elements Yogananda mentions in their work on themselves, plus do psychotherapy work if and when necessary.

6

The Means and Goals Confusion

If our *only* problem was that the boundaries and the splitting that are 'simply' part of the world of matter find their concrete human expression – and possibly a pathological amplification – in the birth process, we might just manage. Then we could build societies and cultures where the shared aim between people could be the move towards unity, towards God. Such societies have existed in the past, but now the dominant world culture is different. Splitting and fragmentation have become the motors of the world. We, as human beings, have the ability to *apply* the process of splitting (ahamkara) that has created us, in the creation of our human environment, thus amplifying the splitting process. The paradox is that underneath massive fragmentation and splitting there lies almost total global inter-dependence, almost like a reflection of universal unity.

Let us now look at another level of these processes that have created this present world, and such confused consciousness in people. The confusion is between means and goals, and a global drama is unfolding on its basis. This process also has a direct effect on the way in which our external world is split and fragmented – a mirror image of the inner world.

Erich Fromm, a psychoanalyst with a strong spiritual leaning, paints a picture of our world in which hedonism has become the accepted norm:

> The Great Promise of Unlimited Progress – the promise of domination of nature, of material abundance, of the greatest happiness for the greatest number, and of unimpeded personal freedom – has sustained the hopes and faith of the generations since the beginning of the industrial age. ... We were on our way to becoming gods, supreme beings who could create a second world, using the natural world only as building blocks for our new creation.[41]

The promise became the main driving force of bourgeois capitalism, and has led to an ever-increasing emphasis on seeking the satisfaction of sense-desires. Fromm defines the two main psychological premises of the industrial system as '(1) that the aim of life is happiness, that is, maximum pleasure, defined as the satisfaction of any desire or subjective need a person may feel (radical hedonism); (2) that egotism, selfishness, and greed, as the system needs to generate them in order to function, lead to harmony and peace'.[42] The point is, it does not have to be like this. Actually, before the industrial revolution maximum pleasure was not considered the main aim in life. Now it has become the driving force of most of our systems, and capitalism needs it for growth, which means more production, more consumption, more pleasure-seeking, discovering new pleasures, but always under the threat of unhappiness, because without that threat the desperate striving for the opposite would not be there. That's what the markets need. Splitting and fear have become the foundations of our way of life.

The opposite worldview is presented in the Vedas. The yogic scriptures and many of the other religious scriptures of the world see the world of gross matter as maya, the world of delusion and duality, where ultimate fulfilment and bliss are not possible. We are here to learn our karmic lessons. The spiritual path of yoga is about withdrawing energy from the senses – the only way out is in – so that the soul can re-connect with God. Capitalism is about exactly the opposite. It needs as much sense orientation in as many people as it can get in order to constantly increase consumption and production. It needs the promise of fulfilment and bliss, and it needs us to fear the opposite. The yogic way on a large scale would be the death sentence for consumerism and capitalism as we know it. It feels as if capitalism *knows* this, and has proceeded to pull spiritual qualities down from the higher realms into consumer goods and pleasure orientation. Greed and envy have become the most important virtues. Yogic wisdom would also say that the greater the pleasure orientation in the world of duality, the greater also the flip side – unhappiness. We seem to be approaching the climax.

In Chapter 7 we are going to use the central model of psychosynthesis to develop a psychospiritual model of alienation, disconnectedness, boundaries and growth- illusion. The model, which I call 'the psychological greenhouse', will draw a psychological map of the world of goods, objects, consumerism, greed and envy. It will be a map of our inner psychological world, which is in a reflective relationship with the outer world. But let us first of all explore how and why capitalism and industrialisation could lead to this world of extreme consumerism and sense-pleasure orientation. Here is a news story.

MODEM MUDDLE KNIFES THE MAC

Eager buyers of Apple's futuristic iMac, the computer with the fashionably frosted blue casing, have discovered that some aspects of it are a tad too futuristic.

Specifically, they have had trouble exploiting its advertised 'plug-straight-in-to-the-internet' capability, because its built-in modem ... actually runs too fast for some telecoms systems. The result: no internet connection.

Other buyers have had problems connecting printers to the iMac, because the printers' manufacturer, Epson, had to scramble to write the software to fit Apple's radical new 'USB' system for connecting gadgets to the £999 iMac. ...

Users also face a Catch-22 in solving the modem problem. Apple's decision to omit a floppy disk drive from the machine means that, although a software 'patch' which tells the modem to run slower, is available, you can only download it from Apple's web site.

But just as the original Catch-22 meant US Airforce pilots could not be excused flying unless they were mad, but wanting to be excused flying meant they were sane, with the iMac you cannot make the connection because of the problems you are having – and if you could make the connection, you wouldn't need the patch.[43]

Situations like the one described in this article are so common nowadays. The complexity of our world makes life difficult in all areas. We really are surrounded by highly interdependent fragments of our own making, constantly trying to correct the errors, conflicts and contradictions that exist between the elements. There is no easy solution to this. Maya is the world of duality and conflict, and at the level of gross matter we cannot resolve all conflict, because even if we sort out certain conflicts, there will still be more further on, and we will still be left with the ultimate one between ego and soul, or life and death.

But we can try and make sense of some of the aspects of maya, of some of the contradictions and conflicts. That's what science is all about. But then, even science and models often just create a different level of maya – the illusion that once we have analysed something sufficiently, we can understand it and put it together again differently, eradicate its contradictions and make it all good and positive. Medicine and a lot of the psychological and environmental sciences are like that, and they succeed to some extent. How far this 'making it better' works is, at least, debatable. There are many examples where the solutions in one area have created new conflicts in another area, often at a higher or more general level. Examples: mass production of meat and BSE; antibiotics and resistant bacteria; fossil-fuel technology and global warming.

So we need to be careful when using models and theories to explain maya and to illuminate our way through it. I am not going to present models and theories to make maya better, because our way through it is by making 'our self' better.

We are now trying to understand how the inner world of splitting is a reflection of (and vice versa) an outer world full of confusion between means and goals, leading to fragmentation. Splitting and fragmentation run like a thread through both our inner and outer worlds. Later on we shall see how this increases the potential for sense-delusions. We need to remain aware here that we are not trying to work out how to make it better. We are only trying to understand so that we can find our way through (beyond) to a deeper level of truth.

Yogananda refers to something like the 'means-goals-confusion' in *The Science of Religion*:

The family man has to earn money to support his family. He starts a certain business and begins to attend to the details that will make it successful. Now, what often happens after a while? The business goes on successfully and money perhaps accumulates until there is much more than is necessary for the fulfilment of his wants and those of his family.

Now one of two things happens. Either money comes to be earned for its own sake and a peculiar pleasure comes to be felt in hoarding, or it may happen that the hobby of running this business for its own sake persists or increases the more. We see that in either case the means of quelling original wants – which was the end – has become an end in itself: money or business has become the end.

Or it may happen that new and unnecessary wants are created and an effort is made to meet them with 'things'. In any case our sole attention drifts from Bliss (which we, by nature, mistake for pleasure and the latter becomes our end). Then the purpose for which we apparently started a business becomes secondary to the creation or increase of conditions or means. ... To put it briefly: from the original purpose of the business, which was the removal of physical wants, we turn to the means – either to the business itself or to the hoarding of wealth coming out of it – or sometimes to the creation of new wants; and because we find pleasure in these we are swept away into pain, which, as we pointed out, is always an indirect outcome of pleasure.[44]

Activity Theory

The last map was about our inner ego-centred psychological processes of splitting and forming boundaries. At the same time the soul wants to move towards unity, towards re-unification with spirit. We are now extending the map to include the outer world more directly in this, and we will see that the outer process is very similar to the inner process. This is quite different from how in the psychotherapy world important aspects of the outer world, like the environment, are usually excluded or just interpreted in their relevance as inner projections. The opposite usually applies to socio-political theories – there the outer world is seen as causal and the inner world as a product.

We are exploring both inner and outer world with the premise that they are in essence the same in that they are both products of the universal process of creation. This does, however, not mean that psychological or socio- political theories do not contain elements of truth. With this in mind, we shall now explore and learn from activity theory.

The basis for a Marxist approach to psychology is activity theory. At university in West Berlin in the 1970s this was part of our curriculum. And it was exciting and highly stimulating, because it presented a world-view and a psychology that was different and far more humane than their established bourgeois counterparts.

I need to include some reasoning why I am using a theory based in Marxist philosophy in a book that is about soul and spirit. In our Western culture Marxism has a bad name, partly because of misunderstandings, partly because his theories have been abused and misrepresented by many so-called socialist countries. I agree with Erich Fromm that 'Marx's aim was that of the spiritual emancipation of man, of his liberation from the chains of economic determination, of restituting him in his human wholeness, of enabling him to find unity and harmony with his fellow man and with nature'.[45]

Marx's analysis of the workings of capitalist society is particularly relevant today, because it clearly identifies the dynamics by which splitting and fragmentation happen as if by 'natural law'. Marxism is not spiritual in any way. Many philosophers before Karl Marx were certainly much more overtly spiritual. Fromm brings Hegel, whose philosophy Marx claimed to have 'turned around', into the comparison: 'Hegel's philosophy of history presupposes an abstract or absolute spirit, which develops in such a way that mankind is only a mass which carries this spirit, consciously or unconsciously'.[46] Marx assigns far more independence to humans: 'As individuals express their life, so they are. What they are, therefore coincides with their production, both with *what* they produce and with *how* they produce. The nature of individuals thus depends on the material conditions determining their production'.[47] This is fascinating because it explains why Marx is so relevant for our psycho-spiritual map-making. He basically says that human beings have 'free will' and that we can create our own stuff (objects *and* relationships) in this world of matter. Based on this premise Marx then proceeds to analyse the material world that we have created and that forms the world into which we are born. This is not dissimilar to the yogic philosophy which emphasises that God has given us 'free will' and that most of the nasty things in our world are caused by us abusing our power of co-creation, our free will.

In Marxist tradition, activity theory is both historical and scientific. It painstakingly analyses the relationships between subject and object in the organic and non-organic world. It then focuses on the process of interaction between living beings and their objects, ultimately the interaction of human beings with their environment. The development of human consciousness is then seen as an evolutionary and historical process, which leads to the splits, contradictions and alienation of class society. The theory explains the historical and societal development of boundaries by seeing their causes in our concrete dealings with our environment. The relationship between the individual and the object is what changes both the individual and the object; internal and external changes in both are a result of their interaction.

Any appreciation of activity theory will need to take into account the fact that it was developed in the 1950s, a time when 'real socialism' was still thriving as a viable alternative to capitalism, and when the damage caused by overpopulation and massive exploitation of planetary resources were not yet obvious. It was this unawareness of planetary ecological issues that allowed both capitalism and socialism to be based on the assumption of continuous growth of resources and productivity to satisfy the ever increasing needs of increasing numbers of people. Well, we now know differently, and we know that both socio-economic systems have with equal ignorance of ecological considerations contributed to global warming, pollution and ozone holes.

However, we need to keep in mind a more general limitation of this theory. The following quote from a book that was published in 1948 addresses this:

> An economic readjustment and equal distribution of the commodities of life cannot be achieved on the basis of the doctrine that pleasure is the chief good in life. The utilitarian philosophy of the greatest pleasure for the greatest number sounds very well, yet it doesn't give any real basis for a man to sacrifice his pleasure for the happiness of another.
>
> Superficial thinkers can find a certain kind of remedy in humanism and Marxian and utilitarian philosophy for existing inequality. They may temporarily remedy certain economic and social evils, but they cannot reach the life of man. Unless his inner life is changed, conflicts and frustration will always remain.[48]

How true this statement has proved to be if we consider the recent demise of the Soviet Union and the Eastern European socialist states.

ACTIVITY AS THE BASIC UNIT OF LIFE

Activity theory says that the psyche and consciousness are a result, a reflection, of the interaction between the individual organism and his environment. The inner world can only be understood in its historical, phylogenetic and ontogenetic relationship with the outer world. The mediator between inner and outer worlds is activity; activity changes the object of the action as well as the subject. The properties of the objective outer world become crystallised in the psyche as reflections gained through active dealings with the objects. As reflections mediated through activity they contain elements of both object and subject, and are therefore never purely objective nor purely subjective. Hence, whatever we think, feel, or do, connects us with our own history and with the history of the world around us. Separateness and isolation become an illusion.

Through activity we modify the environment and the process modifies us. Future generations are then, as we were, born into an environment modified by human activity. We then have to internalise (learn) the modifications that have gone on before us, and proceed to further modify both ourselves and the environment. This model sees historical and personal development, the characteristics of object and subject, as totally interdependent processes, mediated through activity and learning (which is an activity in itself).

We can use any human skill to illustrate the point. Say, someone wants to become a car mechanic now. First of all, in order to have the wish to become a car mechanic, cars and car mechanics must already exist. Even just the wish already connects the person with a large chunk of human history and technical development. Then comes the learning of theories and skills. The connectedness with everything that has gone on before in the history of car-engineering becomes more concrete. Learning also requires language, teachers, books. This connects with other areas of human historical development, like teacher-training, the history of language, of written words, of printing. And so it goes on. Ultimately there are no boundaries between anything, just a gigantic web of inter-action spreading across people and time. But we can be sure that the person who wants to become a car-mechanic would not be conscious of all those inter-connections. With this example we can begin to sense the great paradox that activity theory tries to explain. It is alienation. Increasing complexity and inter-connectedness go hand-in-hand with increasing separation and unconsciousness. Activity theory calls this the split between objective meaning and personal sense. And it is exactly this split that has further cemented boundaries in our conscious-ness, and that can be so skilfully abused.

CONSCIOUSNESS – SENSE AND NONSENSE

The following story is taken from Ben Elton's book *Gridlock* (1991), and illus-trates our fragmented reality. In his 'Off-Planet Introduction' he describes a spaceship hovering above Earth, and the observations the occupants of the vessel are making about our world:

This spaceship contained a group of television researchers from the Planet Brain in the process of analysing humanity, in order to compile a three-minute comedy item for their top-rated television show, That's Amazing, Brainians, which followed the early evening news.

The researchers were pleased, they had noted much which was amusingly amazing, and they assured each other that Earth had provided the easiest bit of researching they had done in aeons. Brain is populated by beings of immense intelligence and so far it had taken them only a quarter, of a quarter, of a single second to assimilate and comprehend humanity.

But then they were stumped. They had encountered one aspect of human activity which astonished and mystified even those hardened researchers. Researchers who thought they had seen every illogicality and lunacy that the universe had to offer. On this very planet they had seen pointless wars and pointless destruction. But this one had thrown them. This one had them scratching their multiple thought podules in a perplexed manner and saying 'akjafgidkersh lejhslh hei !', which translates as 'Bugger me, that's weird !' The problem was one of transport. The Brainians could see the long, thin arteries along which the humans travelled. They noted that after sunrise the humans all travelled one way and at sunset they all travelled the other. They could see that progress was slow and congested along these arteries, that there were endless blockages, queues, bottle-necks and delays causing untold frustration and inefficiency. All this they could see quite clearly.

What was not clear to them, was why. They knew that humanity was stupid, they had only to look at the week's top ten grossing movies to work that out, but this was beyond reason. If, as was obvious, space was so restricted, why was it that each single member of this strange life-form insisted on occupying perhaps fifty times its own ground surface area for the entire time it was in motion – or not in motion, as was normally the case?[49]

Cars and our modes of transport serve as an example here. Other examples could be pollution and other destructive and self-destructive activities that we engage in. Can it make sense? What is the meaning of it? The simple answer to the car situation would be 'Well, we all want cars, big ones, small ones, fast ones, shiny ones, bigger than .... ones'. But why do we all want cars? Status symbol, toy, mode of transport, comfort, needing to get from A to B, speed, no other transport available. All this still does not answer our why-question, because there seem to be too many reasons for having cars, and not one of them relates to congested inner cities, polluted air, and injuries and deaths on the roads. From the spaceship high up in the sky we might see it; down here on Earth we see it differently – we experience the strain and the frustrations of motoring, but this is all made up for by the satisfaction of all those other needs, or so we think. After all, those needs for status and speed, for comfort and individuality are all much more directly personal than some 'high-flying' ideals about a clean and unpolluted environment. We can fool ourselves because we have managed to remove ourselves from our natural environment, and can only see the artificial one that we have created. The artificial environments are created, create and are maintained and expanded by artificial needs and motives. The increasing complexity of our man-made environment blocks off more and more of the natural environment underneath and beyond it.

Here is another nicely written example.

From Mondays to Fridays, most people assume that nature is simply a mechanistic inanimate system; the world is a storehouse of natural resources to be exploited by man as he sees fit for human profit. However, at weekends and especially on holidays, most people revert to a quite different attitude to nature. On Friday evenings, the roads leading out of the great cities of the Western world are clogged as millions of people try to get back to nature in a car. ... A lot of people for example want to get rich, if necessary by exploiting the natural world, causing appalling damage to the environment so they can buy a beautiful place in the country surrounded by acres of unspoilt nature to get away from it all. ... I think that we have to face up the fact that the 9-5 / Monday to Friday attitude is one of the principal causes of the ecological crisis at the present time.[50]

Activity theory sees the historical origins of the split between sense and meaning in the development of tools and in the division of labour. I would say that the origins go further back to the creation of the world of duality and matter itself. But tools and division of labour have speeded up the process. Perhaps this is the point where Marx got it wrong, because of his exclusion of spirituality. Marxist theory states that the people who suffer most from alienation in society, i.e. the working class, are also the ones who deep down carry the need for de-fragmentation and unification. No doubt, this may be true to some extent. But it does not take into account that splitting and the creation of boundaries is a process that is far more deeply ingrained – a characteristic of matter itself that cannot be remedied by social changes, however massive and well-meaning they are. The only part of us that really craves unity is the soul. Marxism tried to see this craving in the ego. We may criticise the socialist systems that used to exist in East Germany and in the Soviet Union for not having applied Marxist theory properly. This is only part of the truth. But for our map-making and sense-making here I should like to use the failure of those systems to emphasise again that the only way out is in – to soul. Otherwise, left within the realms of the ego, the tendency to split and to fragment will just go elsewhere. Corruption, secret service excesses, envy, greed within social structures were rampant in the socialist states. Perhaps recent history just wants to remind us that paradise on Earth is just not on.

There may be an even more essential flaw in Marxist theory. It certainly emphasises the creative potential that is in conflict and contradiction. A revolution, according to Marx, occurs at the point when a conflict between two forces, for example the bourgeoisie and the proletariat, reaches breaking point. In this sense Marxism is similar to the immanent approaches in spirituality and in certain forms of psycho-spiritual self-development. They assume that conflict, emotional turmoil needs to be gone into (experienced) in order to achieve release (revolution) and to then open the heart (the perfect state). It doesn't seem to work like this. I think we can only see and realise the potential in any of the conflicts of the world of duality if we approach them from a soul-perspective. Such a soul-perspective will also lead us to right action.

> ... from the calm center of Bliss you will ultimately learn to disown your own petty desires and to feel only those which seem to be urged in you by a great law.[51]

Going inside before coming out is needed, otherwise it will turn into yet another rainbow chase. The examples for what seeing potential in conflict or in any of our creations can lead to, are many. Nuclear power, genetic engineering, psychotropic medication, fascism are all creations to solve conflicts. We know the devastating effects of some of these revolutionary solutions.

However, what Marxist activity theory does explain is the paradoxical processes of splitting and growing interdependence taking place at the same time. With the development of tools there came increasing division of labour, and the increasing development of systems of co-ordinated actions. To date this paradox, expressed in the example of cars earlier, seems to have reached its peak: society and the activities of groups and individuals in it are extremely separate and, at the same time, totally interdependent. What used to be subordinate operations have now taken on the properties of motivators and have thus created new needs. Personal sense and objective meaning of an activity are often light-years apart; people do different things and are often unaware of the connection between, say a coal-miner and the secretary in a computer software firm, between a psychotherapist and a gardener. Individuality has turned into separation and has become one of the main driving forces behind 'progress'.

What we are facing are different levels of alienation. This alienation is from the collective, and it has been necessary for progress. Using the Marxist activity theory map we can detect different levels of human alienation. These different levels of alienation affirm and strengthen boundaries and fragmentation in our consciousness, which we ultimately need to transcend if we want to re-unite our soul with God.

Alienation

The concept of alienation is central in Marxist theory. It is used to emphasise our alienation from the process of production and consumption, which is created by the 'relationship of production', i.e. the capitalist system. Marx assumed that the workers were the ones who would experience the alienation from the products they produce most strongly, and would therefore change the conditions through a revolution.

For our purposes here it may be useful to look at alienation as the extreme results of splitting and fragmentation, or as manifestations of the means-and-goals confusion. But at the same time we need to keep in mind that alienation carries within itself the potential for unity consciousness. The pattern here might be similar to what we see happening in quantum physics, where the exploration of the smallest particles is leading to revelations about the structure of the universe. Psychologically it may correspond to the fact that we often have to 'hit rock bottom' before we can see the whole picture. Behind it all is the dance between the two great universal forces of attraction and repulsion, of Purusha and Prakruti.

DIVISION OF LABOUR ALIENATION

Division of labour and the development of tools have created a situation where subordinate tasks and goals acquire the quality of being motivational and need satisfying in themselves. This is the basis for the means-and-goals-confusion. In a way the objects of the activity create the need. For example, the production of stamps is only a small part of the overall postal services. However, someone might be extremely motivated to design stamps, while at the same time not being interested in postal services at all. And someone else might be collecting stamps for their colourful images or because they are easier to store than, say, sports-cars, or because there are so many of them available. However, at some level the communication potential between distant people and places forms the overall context even for the production and the collecting of stamps. But we might not be aware of that overall context.

LANGUAGE ALIENATION

The development of language has lead to the separation of the practical from the intellectual. Even though language has developed in close connection with practical activity, it has become, or seems to have become quite independent as 'mental activity'. Jobs can be divided into the two groups of those which require mainly manual skills and those which require mainly intellectual skills. The fact that nowadays intellectual skills are rated more highly than manual ones is leading to divisions and separation between people and to economic illusions. The positive result of this separation (boundary) is all the creations that the human intellect has produced – books, theories, models, philosophies. Intellectual activity has reached the potential to step outside the manual level of activities and be an 'observer' of those levels.

FINANCE ALIENATION

The division between production and finance is what Marx saw as the ultimate capitalist perversion. With the development of money as a means of exchange, trade has become simpler, and human labour could be turned into a commodity with a money value attached to it. Money has become an equaliser between different products, different activities, different people and nations. Regardless of what someone does or has, the money value attached to each object and activity allows comparisons of everything with everything else. The snag is that, in order for it to work, everything needs to have such a value, even time. 'Time is money', hence it can become 'high quality time', 'valuable time', 'useless time', 'time wasted'. This is the basis on which money began to develop a life of its own: the money market, finance capital, interest rates, loans, profits, exchange rates, devaluation etc. Today when we hear about 'the economy' we hear about share indexes, money supply rates, the money market. The interest we get on our deposit account bears for us no conscious relationship to the production side of the economy, but rather with the activities of the 'money markets'. The positive aspect here is the potential for global interchange and comparisons.

COMMUNICATION ALIENATION

Mass communication has created yet another level of alienation. It produced means for communicating selectively and symbolically. The content of a message has become much less important than the way in which it is delivered. The term 'symbolic politics' could be used to describe the end result. Politics is changing; symbols and symbolic actions are increasingly taking the place of what we used to call politics. They are replacing disputes, public choices and political decisions. Symbolic politics always emerges where politics cannot change anything, or where it cannot meet the expectations it has created. Sound bites, spin doctors, PR firms dominate our media culture. It is difficult to see the potential in this aspect of alienation, which is similar to the way advertising uses communication. Perhaps the potential lies in the possibility of reducing the increasing floods of information to shorthand elements – a kind of 'summarising' function.

INTERNET ALIENATION

The world-wide web has created enormous potential for alienation as well as for instant communication and information. The addictive qualities of internet pornography and unreal communication in chat rooms are well known. E-mail communication has created expectations of instant responses and is reducing 'thinking time' before reacting. However, the potential for connecting with people, sites and services all over the planet is fascinating and can be used for the growth of global consciousness. At the same time it may distract from the fact that this global and even universal inter-connection is really only possible at a soul level.

As a result of these processes of alienation on a global scale most individuals cannot see themselves any more as parts of the whole. Greater interdependence has lead to greater individualism, and individualism often means isolation and fragmentation. The alienation of the individual from the context of his activities and his life, as a result of the above stages of alienation, has led to enormous differentiation and expertise. But it has also prepared the ground for rigid boundaries between individuals, between individuals and groups, between groups and nations. The effects of those boundaries as 'battle lines' are competition, domination, 'power over', mistrust etc. However, underneath and beyond all this is growing interdependence between individuals, groups and nations. I see a whole world as just having left the struggles of the BPM 3 state, and rather than moving towards the interdependence issues of BPM 4, trying to apply the rules of 'struggle' from the previous state to the new one. The potential for union and partnership is there. However, as I have expressed earlier, I do not think that the positive potential in any of these societal complexities can be realised without aligning the individual will to the universal will (God's will) first.

Fragmented Objects

There is a system on this planet that has understood how to make use of and benefit from our alienation, our means-and-goals confusion, our muddled boundaries and our craving for unity. That system is systematically using the fragmentation within and without; and it has been using it so successfully that it is now governing large parts of our inner and outer world. It has also begun to fragment and objectify our spiritual craving to such an extent that objects of

FIG. 1: SPLITTING

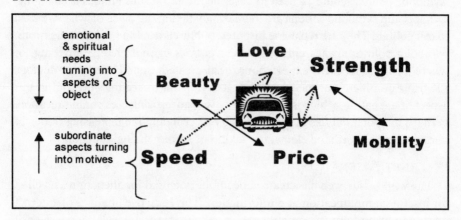

matter have become our Gods. That system itself has grown out of our confused boundary state. The system is consumerism or capitalism and it dominates our lives. Let us continue to draw our map by understanding a system which spreads like a cancerous growth in our consciousness.

Coming back to cars. The initial motive for building cars was as a means of transport, getting from A to B, increased mobility. Since then the simple concept of car has been split up into lots of different cars – the flashy car, the fast car, the big car, the safe car, the environmentally friendly car. Each one of those different cars (or aspects of CAR) has acquired its own set of motives and needs, and more needs have arisen out of this split. For example, mobility and speed have become needs in their own right, quite independent of needing to get from A to B for a particular reason. However, all these different needs are connected to a set of basic emotional needs which are often unconscious. The advertising industry has developed the skills and the methodology to link particular aspects of cars with the underlying, often unconscious, emotional needs and to address them. It has thus become an aim in production and marketing to split a product up into as many different aspects as possible in order to speak to as many different emotional needs as possible. For example – the need for 'newness' means that from time to time products are re-packaged, re-named, re-branded.

Fig. 1 shows how easily an object can be split and how the different aspects of the object (below the line) can become connected with emotional and spiritual needs (above the line). The advertising industry has developed very sophisticated ways of splitting objects and connecting split-off parts with deep emotional and spiritual needs. In the car example, the initially subordinate aspects, like speed, price and mobility, acquire the character of an independent motive; they are promoted to objects in their own right. At the same time spiritual and emotional qualities, like love, beauty and strength, that initially have nothing to do with car, become attached to some of those subordinate aspects. For example, the more expensive car is more beautiful; cars are being advertised using images that stimulate the human need for love and strength. Those emotional/spiritual qualities are thus demoted to objects.

The increasing variety of objects and part-objects created by humanity means that we have become increasingly surrounded by 'things' and these things are often connected with deep inner needs. The satisfaction of those deep inner needs then turns into the need for possession of the objects best representing fulfilment of the emotional needs. We become caught up in the vicious circles of need-wanting-consuming objects etc. Marx wrote that production not only creates the object for the need, but also the need for the object. All this happens with ever increasing numbers of objects competing for the satisfaction of limited numbers of emotional needs. We are caught up in the 'consumer society'.

> We feel that pleasure is something that is intrinsically lacking in the present situation, and that we must manufacture it by surrounding ourselves with sophisticated toys and gadgets. This reinforces the illusion that happiness and pleasure can be piped from the outside, an illusion which itself is responsible for blocking pleasure, so that we end up striving for that which prevents our own joy.[52]

Production also gets pulled into this system: items are invented and produced solely in order to create more variety (e.g. fashion, electric razors). On the consumption side this system then brings out the shadow side of human nature. Extreme expressions of this are greed, theft, envy, eating disorders, addictions, shoplifting etc.

However, this complex system ultimately leaves the emotional needs unsatisfied. From the system's point of view this is a good thing, because it leaves it with lots of 'hungry' consumers. At the same time it has turned people in the industrialised world into human beings who project the satisfaction of their emotional and spiritual needs onto external objects. Emotional and spiritual needs can become 'objectified' to such an extent that people are not aware of the original needs any more. They are only expressed in the need for consumption. Results are attitudes like 'I want more, greater, bigger things', 'I need to work harder, achieve more things', 'I need to be better than others', 'I need to work, produce more efficiently', 'I need to communicate more quickly' – in short, the 'rat-race'. However, apart from creating permanent hunger and craving, the needs expressed in these attitudes are becoming increasingly difficult to satisfy. As a result competition is growing between individuals, groups, companies and nations.

TRUTH OR NOT? (REFLECTION 5)

The 'means-and-goals-confusion' and the associated 'alienation' is making it increasingly difficult for us to make sense of the world we live in, and consequently of our own position and role in this world. This confusion is probably most apparent in the world of politics and the media – contradictory opinions, policies, all containing elements of 'reality' and 'truth', fill political life and time and pages in the mass media.

As an experiment reflect on the following statements:

- *It's difficult enough to keep the economy going, without having to worry about the state of the planet.*
- *Producing more and buying more are important to earn the money to pay for health care and environmental protection.*
- *Progress means having more, knowing more, producing more, needing more and now, producing faster, communicating more quickly.*
- *The whole essence of industrialised society is anti-ecological. Industrial progress means nothing but to process nature bit by bit.*
- *Humanity is in the process of turning the world into one huge production and consumption plant.*

How can you ascertain the truth in each one of those statements? Which ones feel right, which ones wrong, and why? How do you 'make sense' of the world you live in?

KNOWLEDGE AND AWARENESS (REFLECTION 6)

We are all faced with a lifetime and a world where we cannot know everything and where we cannot have everything. We are also increasingly faced with a world where there is so much more to know, so much more to have. In this reflection you are asked to explore the personal implications of this situation.

A. *This first part aims at giving you a sense of the way in which the world of human objects and activities is connected with your personal history and with the history of humanity.*

Pick a human-made object from your present environment. Explore the details of the object with your five senses. Be also open to the other human senses that you experience in the exploration of the object.

As you are exploring the object, you may experience thoughts, feelings, and flashes of memories in relation to this object or other related (or unrelated!) objects. Allow these sensations to be part of your exploration of the object.

Now bring to your conscious mind what you know about the history and the production of the object:

1. *How is the object produced? What are the different stages of its production?*
2. *Imagine the people and their skills that go into the production of the object.*
3. *What is the history of the object, and of the people who are making it? What are the human emotions that you can sense in the history?*
4. *Now imagine all the people who are using the object. Where would it be used and who would use it? What emotions do you sense in the users of the object?*

B. *Now select an object or an activity that you know little about but that you would like to know more about. Explore your thoughts and feelings connected with this.*

Then imagine that in this lifetime you will not be able to know everything about that object or activity. What does that feel like?

This part of the reflection will probably get you in touch with your one-pointed, focused mind – the mind that puts energy into acquiring knowledge and skills. It may also stimulate the frustration and helplessness of the realisation of your limitations. Be with those feelings for a few moments.

Reflection 6 shows that for most objects it is unlikely that we have sufficient knowledge to be able to trace their history accurately. However, part A of the exercise aims at giving you a sense of the connectedness of the world of knowledge, emotions, individual and collective history. Sensing this ultimate connectedness behind the complexity and fragmentation can begin to open our hearts. It is a way of sensing unity behind the fragments, but it is not the way to cosmic unity consciousness, because for that we have to go inside first. You can feel united with the whole world and still be disconnected from God. However, you are more likely to find God once you start seeing units rather than fragments.

Part B in Reflection 6 hints at how the limitations and frustrations in striving for the potentially endless acquisition of knowledge and things can dominate your mental activity. This is the path of the 'hungry customer' that is promoted so much in our culture. It is a path that ultimately keeps you away from awareness and wisdom. It is a path that promotes the intellect in favour of soul-intelligence.

7

The Psychological Greenhouse

Both psychoanalysis and Marxist activity theory analyse splitting and fragmentation in our inner and outer worlds. Even though the theoretical frameworks of the approaches would see themselves as very different, the patterns they discover are remarkably similar. For the spiritually minded yogi this does not come as a surprise. Neither would it come as a surprise for many of the modern cosmologists, nuclear physicists and quantum theorists. It is the same patterns and processes that permeate the world of gross matter, the world of maya, including our conscious and subconscious mind.

Can you sense the dilemma that is creeping in between the lines? You may ask: What then is the point in trying to improve things, trying to make it all better? If conflict, contradictions, splitting and fragmentation are an integral part of the whole show, why then spend years in psychotherapy to become a reasonably reasonable person? Why then spend all this time and energy trying to help others, trying to fight for good causes? Answer: Because right action is part, but only part, of trying to get through the inner and outer clouds of fragmented matter that fill us and surround us. But we must not think that it can all be resolved through right action. The other part of breaking through the clouds is the going inside, going beyond, transcending. From that point right action becomes non-attached right action.

Let us now move on to a map, which pulls the previous ones together by incorporating elements of both inner and outer world considerations. It is an expansion of the basic model of psychosynthesis, which was developed by the Italian psychiatrist Roberto Assagioli. The map will show how extreme the situation is, how disconnected from spirit we really are, and how we need to break through the dark clouds that surround us – through our inner and outer pollution.

Psychosynthesis is a school of psychotherapy that calls itself psycho-spiritual. That means that it differs from most other schools, and there are many, in that it explicitly, in its models and in its therapeutic approach, includes the notions of spirit and soul. People are seen as spiritual beings, and in psychosynthesis psychotherapy the client is not only seen as a struggling individual, but also as a soul on a journey.

However, our map-drawing will go beyond psychosynthesis. Having trained and worked as a supervisor in psychosynthesis for many years, I now feel that psychosynthesis, like other transpersonal psychotherapies, can be confused with a 'spiritual path'. But it can only be a possible stepping stone towards a spiritual path, because the models lack certain spiritual elements which, I think, are vital for the journey inside. I know that some of my colleagues may disagree with me. They may think that psychosynthesis and other transpersonal therapies offer sufficient spiritual impetus to clients to enable them to engage in a spiritual discipline if appropriate for them. My concern, however, is that psychospiritual therapies can actually confuse clients and trainees into thinking that they are on a spiritual path and thus prevent them from finding proper spiritual teachings and discipline. My concerns here are similar to the ones I expressed earlier in the critique of the BPM model and we shall use those concerns later to develop the psychosynthesis model further. With this in mind, let us now appreciate a two-dimensional map derived from psychosynthesis.

Assagioli writes about the spiritual elements of our personality:

[They] come down like rays of sunlight into the human personality – into our personal consciousness – and form a link between our ordinary human personality and the spiritual 'I', the spiritual Reality. They are like rays of light pouring down, taking on various shades of colour and dispersing, depending on the permeability or the transparency of our personal consciousness. ... everything that exists externally, in concrete form and individually is the manifestation, effect and reflection of a higher, transcendent, spiritual Reality. ...

This indeed is the secret: to recognise that external things have no true value, significance or reality of their own, that they only serve to highlight or represent inner realities and spiritual qualities.[53]

The Egg Diagram

So far our maps have not really been proper maps, i.e. diagrammatic, mainly two-dimensional representations of reality. This is changing now and we are starting off with the first drawn map of the psyche, a two-dimensional one that will later grow into a three-dimensional one.

The most important chart in psychosynthesis is the 'egg diagram'. It is a map that contains the most important elements of our psyche in a schematic way. A version of it is represented here, and I shall use it to develop some ideas about the psycho-spiritual implications of consumerism. The following descriptions of the areas of consciousness, as illustrated overleaf in Fig. 2 (The Egg Diagram), are taken from Assagioli's book *Psychosynthesis*.[54]

(1) The **lower unconscious** contains 'the elementary psychological activities which direct the life of the body; the intelligent co-ordination of bodily functions;

FIG 2: THE EGG DIAGRAM

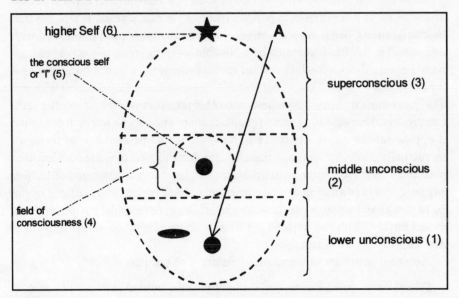

the fundamental drives and primitive urges; many complexes, charged with intense emotion; dreams and imaginations of an inferior kind; lower, uncontrolled para-psychological processes; various pathological manifestations, such as phobias, obsessions, compulsive urges and paranoid delusions.'

(2) The **middle unconscious** 'is formed of psychological elements similar to those of our waking consciousness and easily accessible to it. In this inner region our various experiences are assimilated, our ordinary mental and imaginative activities are elaborated and developed in a sort of psychological gestation before their birth into the light of consciousness.'

(3) The **higher unconscious** or superconscious: 'From this region we receive our higher intuitions and inspirations – artistic, philosophical or scientific, ethical 'imperatives' and urges to humanitarian and heroic action. It is the source of the higher feelings, such as altruistic love; of genius and of the states of contemplation, illumination, and ecstasy. In this realm are latent the higher psychic functions and spiritual energies.'

(4) The **field of consciousness** is the 'the incessant flow of sensations, images, thoughts, feelings, desires, and impulses which we can observe, analyse, and judge.'

(5) The **conscious self** or 'I' is the point of pure self-awareness, not to be confused with the personality. The changing contents of our consciousness (the sensations, thoughts, feelings etc.) are one thing, while the 'I', the self, the centre of our consciousness is another. The 'I' is the centre of pure self awareness, the place that the psychosynthesis disidentification exercise leads to. It is also the first stage of detachment that can be reached in meditation.

(6) The **higher Self**: The 'I' is a reflection of the higher Self. 'The conscious self … seems to disappear altogether when we fall asleep, when we faint, when we are

under the effect of an anaesthetic or narcotic, or in a state of hypnosis. And when we awake the self mysteriously re-appears, we do not know how or whence … . This leads us to assume that the re-appearance of the conscious self or ego is due to the existence of a permanent centre, of a true Self situated beyond or 'above' it.' Assagioli thus saw the aim of Psychosynthesis: 'What has to be achieved is to expand the personal consciousness into that of the Self; to reach up, following the thread or ray to the star; to unite the lower with the higher Self'. Soul can thus be seen as an energetic experience of a connection between the 'I' and the higher Self.

(7) The **collective unconscious**: The egg diagram is always drawn with dotted lines as its perimeter. This is meant to indicate our interconnectedness at the levels of our psychological being. Each individual consciousness is influenced by, connected with, and influences the 'collective' surrounding it. The collective contains the evolutionary and historically grown, crystallised experiences of humanity and of life on this planet and beyond.

Earlier I quoted Assagioli writing about the 'spiritual elements of our personality that come down like rays of sunlight into the human personality – into our personal consciousness – and form a link between our ordinary human personality and the spiritual 'I', the spiritual Reality'. In the egg diagram I have labelled one of those rays A. They are intuitive flashes, inspirations, 'callings' from the higher realms, in short, energies that help the reconnection of the 'I' and the Self. Sometimes these rays, like ray A, may even be sufficient to transform a complex or a conflict in the lower unconscious.

Objects as Protection

Let us now go back to consumerism. Essentially human beings have to produce and consume in order to stay alive. Goods and objects can be seen as protecting the ego from the survival and annihilation fears of the lower unconscious. Many of the childhood fears and depressions that lie dormant in the lower regions are related to the child's fear of abandonment, loss of emotional and physical nourishment, and ultimately death. This is the region of the psyche that most psychotherapies delve into. In Fig. 3 I am placing the objects as a protective barrier between the lower unconscious and the middle unconscious. The objects thus stabilise the ego, 'hold it together'.

The objects in the diagram are rather simplified; apart from solid goods there are many 'potential objects'. The huge field of psychoanalytic models and theories applies here, so that ultimately other people, the self-image, feelings and actions can serve as objects that make up the protective barrier. Eventually this barrier can turn into the 'neurotic space', which needs to be constantly filled up in order to protect from the fears and conflicts that are rooted in the subconscious mind. The objects then become interchangeable, and especially in eating disorders

FIG. 3: OBJECTS AS PROTECTION

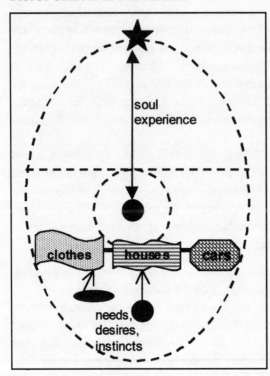

and in addiction the consumption of food and other substances serves this 'filling up' process.

At a different level, the splitting and fragmentation which is caused by the ever increasing division of labour required to produce the ever more detailed parts and components of complex objects (e.g. the components needed to produce a car), eventually turns activities into objects to fill the space. Thus we could have objects like career, mortgage, DIY skills etc. filling the space as well.

It is obvious how the growth-obsession in our society feeds into this process through the constant need for more objects. Even when the space is full, more objects need to be squeezed into it, because 'grow or die' is the ultimate law. Eventually the process needs new space to fit in more and more objects.

Objects as Distraction

The continuous flow of objects into limited space requires the expansion of the available (psychological) space. Money and finance have reduced many of the objects to a common denominator. Ten one-thousand pound notes require less space than a car, and thus the overriding consideration in society and, to a lesser extent, in our individual psyche has become to 'make money', to have shares, pensions and profits, in short money as a protection from fear and depression. We cannot escape chequebooks, credit cards and 'budgeting' any more. Money has become the main driving force – it needs to be 'made', regardless of how. Money has created a market for itself – the world's economies are run according to the rules of those markets. The most important rule is that money needs to grow; interest rates, investment, stocks, bonds, pension funds – they all assume that a certain amount of money 'grows' to a larger amount. The growth of money happens as if by natural law.

Money has become the main driving force, and consumption and production have been demoted to subordinate elements; consumption and production are equalised and are measured with the yardstick 'money'. Money itself has become a commodity, and a quality that is attached to goods – the expensive car, the expensive house. Hence production and consumption have become means to make money, and the character, quality and quantity of the goods that are produced and consumed become increasingly irrelevant. In its most abstract expression as shares and speculative capital, money has developed a life of its own. It has become so powerful that it can make or break whole nations and severely influence all our well-being regardless of how much we work, produce and spend.

However, in order to produce more (to make more money), somewhere down the line people need to consume more. Hence growing populations mean growing markets, mean growing consumption. The system has also devised numerous ways to stimulate consumption in the existing markets, advertising and re-packaging have become the motor of the process. The neurotic space becomes overcrowded with objects in colourful wrappings.

As the lower barrier has become more solid, making many people especially in the Western world feel well protected, the space needs to be widened. New motives for producing and consuming have to be created. And the new motives are increasingly found in the higher realms. Figure 1 on page 84 illustrates how subordinate aspects of the object 'car' can become connected with unconscious emotional needs. We are now going one step further by saying that this applies to needs from the lower unconscious as well as the higher unconscious. The expansion of marketing and advertising has meant that increasingly qualities and motives from the higher realms have become associated with products. As a result the upper border of the middle unconscious with the higher unconscious is also becoming filled up with objects, or with aspects of objects. It is as if the higher qualities were pulled down from the higher realms, creating an objectified spiritual space, a reflection of the lower neurotic space. At the same time qualities from the lower unconscious are being promoted by attaching them to the higher qualities. (See Fig. 4.)

FIG. 4: OBJECTS AS DISTRACTION

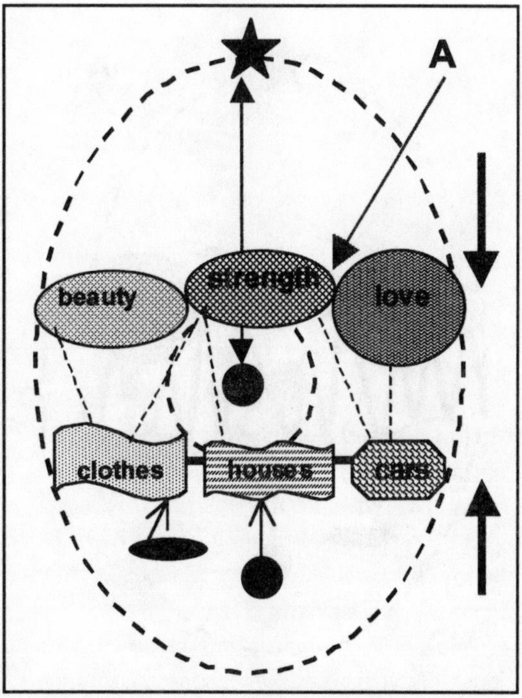

An additional complication arises from the fact that some of the higher qualities carry in themselves the desire to 'own' them and are therefore particularly
prone to this process. Assagioli writes about 'beauty':

> On the one hand we can say that among the attributes of God beauty is the
> most easily recognisable because it is the one first manifested in ancient
> times, the most tangible attribute, one that left its imprint in concrete, mate-
> rial forms, and the attribute that struck the senses and the imagination
> more directly than any other. On the other hand it is clearly the most
> dangerous attribute, one that more than any other ties man to matter and
> form, and one which more than any other produces in him the desire for
> sensory pleasure, the sense of selfish, separate ownership, an attribute that
> more than any other blinds and deceives man, enveloping him in the irides-
> cent veils of Maya – those of the Great Illusion – and thus the attribute
> which most distances him and keeps him separate from God, the deep
> Reality of Truth. … Because beauty is the divine quality that has assumed
> the most concrete expression, has been made tangible and manifested itself
> in matter, it is the one man can most readily abuse, without recognising its
> noble origin. The quality of beauty is no longer related to its source, rather
> it has come to be regarded as a quality that resides in matter itself and in
> its concrete forms.[55]

FIG. 5: THE PSYCHOLOGICAL GREENHOUSE

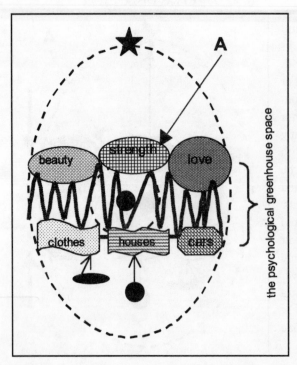

The result is shown in
Fig. 5, where both the
lower and the upper border
of the middle unconscious
are filled up with objects,
aspects of objects, and
reflections of objects. The
space becomes rather
crowded.

Ultimately this situation
turns into what I call the
'psychological green-
house'. We are familiar
with the global greenhouse
effect, where the incoming
heat from the sun gets
trapped by greenhouse
gases in the atmosphere,
thus leading to rising
temperatures and changes
in climates on the earth's

surface. The psychological greenhouse effect is similar in that energies from the higher and the lower realms get trapped in the middle unconscious and in the field of consciousness, thus leading to a 'heating up' of that area. The crowded space also prevents an easy connection between the 'I' and the higher Self, thus making the experience of soul very difficult.

The Greenhouse Psyche

Many of the stressful situations that govern our lives can be seen in those terms: the endless striving for more and more things and satisfaction; the increasing speed with which we need to do and have it all; the 'feeling trapped' and 'no way out'; the inability to step out.

The psychological problems connected with this effect of the psychological greenhouse are all the stress-related conditions that we see ever increasingly around us and within. It is important to note here that these definitions of common stress-related problems do not intend to negate their origins in the dynamics of the lower unconscious, but rather intends to show how the psychological greenhouse is a space where they are amplified rather than resolved, and to some extent caused.

ANXIETY, PANIC, AND STRESS SYMPTOMS

Everything has become too much. Over a long period of overstimulation and striving driven by fear, fear has finally overtaken and the striver is left behind. The gap becomes bigger and fear takes over more and more. Panic attacks triggered by certain stimuli are the body-mind trying to make sense of it all, thus attaching the fear to specific situations. The situations that fear is attached to usually have to do with too much or too many (people, objects in supermarkets, cars on the motorway), too little or too few (open spaces, loneliness) or the inevitability of death (striving leading nowhere).

OBSESSIONAL RITUALS

Children carry out rituals to structure, make sense of, a world that is too complex. People in the psychological greenhouse carry out rituals to create their own safe space, protected from the bombardment of objects. Cleaning and checking rituals, the battle against intrusive thoughts can be seen as the individual's struggle against being taken over by the uncontrollable forces around him. Perfectionism, excessive worrying, inability to make decisions are aspects of our disorientation in the face of a world crowded with people, objects and thoughts, and a lack of spiritual guidance.

SEXUAL PROBLEMS

The one area of human interaction where intimacy and union are possible becomes dominated by performance and competition. The need to dominate over the partner turns people into objects and ultimately their own sexuality into an object as well. Thus 'objectified', sexuality becomes open to 'market forces': it can be split up, different aspects can be turned into objects, money can be made with it, and ultimately our fears of each other and of intimacy can be turned into something marketable rather than something that sexuality can help us overcome.

'Inner sanctuary' or soul can be defined as an energetic experience of a connection between 'I' and Self (see Fig. 2). It happens when the 'I' is energised, infused, 'held' by the Self, rather than by the objects surrounding it. It is an experience of inner calm, stillness, solidity that is not dependent on external circumstances. If, however, the connection between 'I' and Self as in the diagram is blocked, then sanctuary will only be found in the withdrawal into the 'I'. The search for sanctuary can turn into separation, depression, alcoholism, addiction, autism, which are all ways of closing the 'I' off from the hectic activity, the heating-up that goes on around it.

The Potential in the Greenhouse

The danger is that the scale of the economic, ecological, psychological and spiritual disasters overwhelms us, once we begin to see them with heart and soul. As a result we may desperately want to repress our insights again, just to continue in our old sweet ways. Yes, it is nice to believe that there are niches in all the mess; that maybe we will get out of this crisis or the next one and that everything will be OK again; that maybe the Earth can cope with it all. Or we can ask about the potential in the greenhouse. Can we use technology, science, money, wealth in 'the right way'? Is there a right way? Asking those questions is similar to trying to find the potential in alienation, splitting, BPM 3 etc. The answer, as before, is yes *and* no.

When we ask those questions, we are basically trying to make things right; we are trying to see challenges instead of obstacles. Most psychotherapies do just that – turning old destructive patterns into challenges on the path of self-development. But that, again, leaves us muddling around in the world of duality. We resolve conflicts at one level, only to be faced with new ones at a different level. And so it goes on.

One obvious potential of the greenhouse lies in the fact that spiritual qualities are brought down to earth. They are often twisted and abused, but at the same time they are also very close. Michael Lindfield emphasises the potential in information technology:

> The new information technology is bringing about an even more fundamental change: it is the first technology to extend our mental capacity as a species and in effect is an expansion of our brain and nervous system. An increase in mental capacity and logical ability alone will not build the more caring future we so desire. We need a corresponding technology to expand the human heart and increase its capacity to love and care.[56]

In addition to information technology, the same would apply to transport, housing, the media and many of the other 'achievements' of humanity. Could this then be the solution? Could the 'power of the heart' transform the overcrowded, claustrophobic psychological space into something else?

In a more recently published collection of writings entitled *Money and the Spiritual Life*, Assagioli addresses a similar issue. He probably wrote it in 1937 and I should like to quote it here, because I have earlier shown how money and finance capital have increased and alienated the production and consumption of objects.

> More than anything else spirituality is concerned with considering life's problems from a higher, enlightened, synthetic point of view, testing every-thing on the basis of true values, endeavouring to reach the essence of every fact, neither allowing oneself to stop at external appearances nor to be taken in by traditionally accepted views, by the way the world at large looks at things, or by our own inclinations, emotions and preconceived ideas. ... When spiritual light is focused on the most complex of individual and collective problems it produces solutions and reveals ways in which we can avoid many dangers and errors, sparing us much suffering and thus bestowing incalculable benefits on our lives.[57]

In his analysis Assagioli then moves on to use an approach that is quite similar to the one I have used in defining money. He urges us to go back to seeing it as an instrument rather than a goal in itself:

> Thus the first spiritual act we need to perform is to free ourselves from this tendency to place too much value on the means, or on the instrument whereby worldly goods are acquired and exchanged: money. Let us be determined in our refusal to offer any further sacrifices on the altar of this false god, let us free ourselves from the fascination this idol has for us and, with an unclouded vision and calm indifference, reduce it to what it actu-ally is: a mere instrument, a useful device, a practical convention.
> ... The basis for correct individual use lies in the concept of possessions itself as a personal right. Legal ownership is purely a human invention, but one that is justified psychologically and practically in view of the limited level of moral development man has reached. The desire to possess is a primordial force that cannot be discounted: it cannot be killed or forcibly repressed. In spiritual terms, however, ownership has a very different aspect and significance. No longer is it a personal right, but a responsibility towards God and man.
> ... From the spiritual point of view, then, man may only consider himself a trustee, guardian or administrator of the material goods for which he has obtained legal ownership. Those goods are for him a real test, a test he must submit to.[58]

So we are presented with two strategies for turning the greenhouse around.

Assagioli advocates the more analytical approach of 'going back to basics' and then applying spiritual principles to the basic components, while Lindfield suggests the 'seeing with the heart' – the application of qualities like caring, compassion, service, altruism towards the world around us, including ourselves. Other writers and thinkers describe this as the necessary shift in value systems from the masculine to the feminine.

How do these two strategies complement each other or differ from each other? Is one of them the masculine approach and the other the feminine? How does each need the other, and what would that look like in action?

There are plenty of approaches to self-development, therapy and growth that put a lot of energy into the above questions. Impressively creative solutions, workshops, emotional outbursts, 'working through' have been developed to harness the potential in our world of inner and outer crises. However good-willed, helpful and exciting many of these approaches are, we need to be aware of their possible limitations in the same way that we have explored the limitations of psychotherapy, Marxism etc. The yardstick for measuring approaches like these will have to be whether they start off with or include a soul-perspective. Because if we see the psychological greenhouse as an extreme and all-pervading expression of the duality of matter, then our present challenges are not qualitatively different from the ones we have faced since Adam and Eve. Only, perhaps, it is now becoming much clearer that the only way out is in. The psychological greenhouse space is becoming so frantic, addictive, violent, perverse that it is also becoming more difficult to find immanent solutions. Transcendence seems to be required (asked of us?). We are at the same crossroads that we have always been at, but it is as if God has put up a really big, brightly lit signpost.

The signpost is made up of extremes of suffering and extremes of sense-pleasure seeking. Both go hand-in-hand, as we know. We have to choose, because our attachment to seeking sense-pleasures has gone so far that it is draining all life energy out of the spiritual centres in the spine and in the brain. In the greenhouse model this is expressed by the way in which lower energies are *glued* to higher energies. In the section on *The Pendulum*, which will contain one of the final maps for the journey inside, we shall explore what it means when we say that life energy is pulled out of the spiritual centres. For this we shall expand the greenhouse map into a three-dimensional model.

But let us first of all look at the signs more closely, using the maps we have acquired so far.

YOUR INNER GREENHOUSE (REFLECTION 7)

In this reflection I should like you to imagine your own personal psychological greenhouse.

A. *Put a large sheet of paper in front of you and copy the egg diagram onto it. Put yourself right in the middle. At the border between the middle and the lower unconscious write down all the things that you have achieved and created in your life that make you feel safe. Also put down all your most important activities that create for you that feeling of safety and security. Be aware how important those things are for you. Be also aware how much energy and time you have been and are putting into creating this protective wall.*

At the border between the middle and the higher unconscious write down those higher qualities that are connected for you with the objects and activities that you have put down below. You can choose from Maslow's 'values of the consciousness of being', which are:

- *the sense of fulness, integration, totality;*
- *the sense of perfection, completion, vitality and intensity of life;*
- *the sense of richness;*
- *the sense of simplicity;*
- *the sense of beauty;*
- *consciousness of goodness;*
- *absence of effort;*
- *spontaneity;*
- *joy;*
- *cheerfulness;*
- *humour;*
- *the sense of truth;*
- *the sense of independence and inner freedom.*

Also consider qualities like love, altruism, partnership and companionship, in your considerations. The questions you are asking are: How much is my 'sense of richness' connected with my salary'? How much is my 'sense of freedom' linked with the car I have and the holidays I can afford? How much do I express or receive love through the giving and receiving of material goods?

You may find that a lot of your higher qualities are firmly linked with just a few objects or activities. Obviously this could mean that there is great fear for you of losing those objects or activities, because it would mean losing the freedom, joy, love, cheerfulness, beauty in your life.

Spend a few moments reflecting upon your own personal psychological greenhouse. How do you feel right in the middle of it? And imagine what it would be like to have all those higher qualities independent of the objects and activities below. Can you imagine it? What would you really like to do and still have those higher qualities? What would you really like to own and still have those higher qualities? Make notes.

B. *You have now mapped your own psychological greenhouse. Don't worry how well you have done it. The important part is that you are beginning to realise how important objects and activities have become to satisfy your higher needs, and how fear pushes you to do more and more, to own more and more in order to hold on to those higher qualities. Let's move on to the second part of this exercise, which may be rather painful.*

I should like you to consider how much you feel you need to use the following qualities, characteristics, activities, to keep your greenhouse going. Think of your daily life, work and private, and ask yourself how much you feel compelled, by circumstances or otherwise, to use, to experience or to have to put up with each one of the following qualities. Rate each one of the qualities on a scale from 1 to 5 for their relevance for you:

Anger	Boredom	Confusion
Control	Cruelty	Cynicism
Deceit	Destructiveness	Disappointment
Dishonesty	Fear	Force
Frustration	Futility	Greed
Guilt	Hostility	Hypocrisy
Ignorance	Intolerance	Isolation
Jealousy	Manipulation	Miserliness
Misery	Paranoia	Recklessness
Rejection	Revenge	Scarcity
Self delusion	Self importance	Self indulgence
Selfishness	Spite	Stagnation
Stubbornness	Suspicion	Worry

Look at the drawing of your psychological greenhouse and look at those qualities that you have rated 4 and 5. And then reflect on the following questions:

Is this how I want my life to be?

What do I really want in life?

What is really important for me in life?

What are my ideals and values?

C. *With those questions in mind close your eyes and imagine yourself at the centre in your drawing. Imagine that you are asking those questions from deep down in your heart. Feel the energy that those questions have. Then imagine yourself standing on a meadow – feel the ground under your feet. You are looking up and above you can see a thick layer of grey clouds. Now focus all the energy of those questions, deep down from your heart up to the clouds. Your feet are standing solidly on the ground. See how gradually an opening appears*

in the clouds. The sun shines through that opening down on you. Feel the warmth of the
rays as they reach you. There may also be a symbol coming down to you with the rays.

Draw the symbol on the sheet with your greenhouse map.

It is quite scary to see the list of words in the reflection above. They are the demons from a deck of little cards called *the demon cards*, a counterpart of *the angel cards*. They are the human qualities that the greenhouse brings out in us and also needs for its survival. But the greenhouse has not created those qualities. They are part of *evil*, the stuff that Shakespeare's dramas are made of. So, what do we need to do not to get caught up in those energies, not to be swallowed up by them? Where does evil come from and why is it part of our universe?

8

Evil and Wisdom

The psychological greenhouse is ultimately a symptom or expression of the duality of the world of matter. The fragmentation that characterises it is created by the psychological, societal and socio-economical splitting mechanisms that we have discussed. But ultimately, the mechanisms themselves are also an expression of the world of duality. The patterns and the dynamics that create them are similar at all levels and in all areas. And however much we try to find one-ness, bliss, happiness within this world of duality and with the means of this world, we can only find it temporarily. We will always get the flip-side of the coin as well – unhappiness, fear, depression, misery, illness. Our maps have led us to the point of realising the falseness of many of the official maps to fulfilment. What now? Cynical withdrawal from the world certainly seems an attractive option at this stage. However, let us move on with the exploration, because there is a way in which we can achieve happiness, balance and serenity in this world and in this life. It just doesn't work the way we think and the way we are led to believe.

In order to proceed with mapping our way inside we need to really understand and concentrate on something that has been referred to throughout the previous chapters. It is the overstimulation of the senses. The sense orientation of our world and our lives has received a pretty bad press throughout this book. The psychological greenhouse model shows how our sense orientation is amplified, abused, and used as the motor for our capitalist and consumerist culture.

In order to find a very personal and practical way to overcome this core issue in the world of duality we now need to understand the process at a personal level. It is difficult to comprehend how we could possibly go beyond the senses on our path. We can easily understand that sensationalism might not be a good thing. But sense, sensitivity, sensuality – are those not all positive, deeply human characteristics? And what about all our emotions? They are all connected with our mind and our senses. Is the richness of the human emotions not a good thing?

But there is another question that comes out of our journey so far. It is more abstract and, at first sight, appears less personal. It is the question of evil, because all the nasty qualities listed in the greenhouse reflection could be called evil.

Ultimately the consideration of both questions, that of sense orientation and that of evil, will lead to the same point. But the structure of a book, i.e. the two-dimensional sequencing of words and sentences, enforces a certain order, a before and after. This can, at times, feel arbitrary for the reader, and for the writer it poses questions of how to present a sequence of thoughts about something that is not sequential.

The greenhouse considerations have left us with at least those two avenues along which to proceed. I know where I want to get to with my writing. You do not, and I am arguing and exploring on different levels. But I can assure you that all those different levels will lead to the same point. Fig. 6 illustrates this. In the beginning the different levels of seeing, for example the psychological and the socio-economical, appeared quite separate (A). But they appear separate only because we have split them into separate

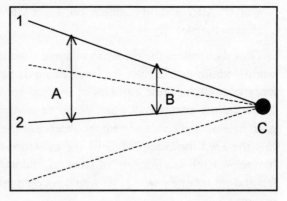

FIG. 6: TOTAL ONE-NESS

things. It is like all the splitting and fragmentation that we have discussed and explored so far. And writing, unfortunately, is very much a splitting process, because it has to use words, sentences, all in a linear sequence. However, reading can be different. For example, Yogananda recommends the following process for reading inspirational texts: read for 15 minutes, reflect on what you have read for thirty minutes, and then meditate for one hour. I am not necessarily suggesting this procedure for this book. But, for example, by using the reflections you can personalise the text and thus go beyond my linear sequence of writing.

Ultimately, when our understanding is beginning to come more from our intuition rather than just the intellect, the differences between things and between levels of seeing become smaller (B) and smaller until they reach the point of total one-ness (C). That is the point from where we can see differences and discrepancies far away in the distance, while our soul can experience the one-ness that is represented by point C.

Good and evil feels like a touchy subject to write about. How can evil be part of creation, part of God's creation? And if we accept it as part of creation, how can we be free of it? Do we need to be free of it? Is this just the way it is? Isn't it just part of our animal nature, part of life? This is exactly what the greenhouse-system would want us to believe. And then the drama in Shakespeare's plays or in Goethe's *Faust* turns the battle between good and evil into entertainment that touches us somewhere, because it reflects some of our own struggles. But we are promoting it to the level of respectable culture, to a night out at the theatre. The same is true for the struggle between good and evil that fills our TV screens and the minds of our children. At some level I agree with Grof:

> The existence of the shadow side of creation enhances its light aspects by providing contrast and gives extraordinary richness and depth to the universal drama. The conflict between good and evil in all the domains and on all the levels of existence is an inexhaustible source of inspiration for fascinating stories. A disciple once asked Sri Ramakrishna, the great Indian visionary, saint, and spiritual teacher: 'Swamiji, why is evil in the world?' After a short deliberation, Ramakrishna replied succinctly: 'To thicken the plot'.[59]

Grof then invites the reader to imagine a world without evil, for example a world without disease. But far from giving us paradise on earth, it would do away with all the great pioneers of medical research, and even with Mother Teresa and her admired activities. Without totalitarian regimes we would lose the great freedom fighters; and with the absence of metaphysical evil we might even lose the need for God. For Grof the existence of evil is responsible for the 'immense depth and richness' of creation, and without it he envisages a colour-less and uninteresting world that would not even provide the material for a movie or a play.

Paramahansa Yogananda often uses the metaphor of a movie to describe maya, the world of delusion, and the contrast between good and evil in this world:

> Without shadows as well as light there could be no picture. Evil is the shadow that converts the one beam of God's light into pictures and forms. Therefore, evil is the shadow of God that makes this play possible.[60]

Here too, the message is not to take the whole show too seriously. But at the same time Yogananda places great emphasis on evil being a test for our free will, a test of whether we choose good or evil.

The entertainment value of the struggle must not distract us from fighting the battle inside, because, according to the science of yoga, that is what we are meant to do.

> The old orthodox way is to deny temptation, to suppress it. But you must learn to control temptation. It is not a sin to be tempted. Even though you are boiling with temptation, you are not evil; but if you yield to that temptation you are caught temporarily by the power of evil. You must erect about yourself protecting parapets of wisdom. There is no stronger force that you can employ against temptation than wisdom. Complete under-standing will bring you to the point where nothing can tempt you to actions that promise pleasure, but in the end will only hurt you.[61]

Much has been written about good and evil since humans began to reflect their existence. Here I would like to present my model, which reflects the way in which I understand Yogananda's teaching on good and evil.

I have no doubt that evil exists as an energy in the world and that we all have good and evil inside. I am also convinced that it is our task, individually and collectively to move from evil to good, or to reduce our evil parts and increase our good parts. I further believe that evil is there so that we *can* move towards good – our relationship with evil is our teacher. But we must also keep in mind that life in the world of duality is only a show, albeit a very dramatic one. What appears to be evil here on this level of existence may well look completely different and have a different function if seen from a few levels further up. Remember the example of the life-maintaining function of earthquakes and volcanoes on p. 38.

There is a pattern in fairy tales and myths which can explain the role of evil on our path. The fairy tale journey often starts off with innocence. But innocence on its own is not complete. Something is missing; it cannot survive like this. Further lessons need to be learned before moving on is possible. The hero then sets out to find the missing part. He has to go through the darkness, fight monsters, risk his own life in order to find that missing part. He has to go through evil, darkness, the shadow. To find what? The *what* does not seem to be as important as the trials on the journey itself. The hero usually returns a different person, with more compassion, heart, and with wisdom. The object he set out to find has lost its relevance, but he has found something within himself – his heart or soul – that allows him to overcome the initial problem. This represents our inner journey.

Fig. 7 illustrates the journey from *innocence* to *heart*. It is similar to the journey from BPM 1 to BPM 4. *Evil* provides us with the tests and trials on our life path, so that we can end up in our *heart* (compassion, transpersonal love, soul). It is, of course, possible to get stuck in the darkness, or to spend long periods of time there. The grey areas where innocence overlaps with evil, and where heart overlaps with evil, are particularly dangerous and confusing. They are the areas of *abuse* and *addiction*. Confusion arises because sometimes both, abuse and addiction, can feel as if they were belonging to Innocence or Heart. It is also these areas of addiction and abuse that are often used by the greenhouse system.

FIG. 7: THE JOURNEY FROM INNOCENCE TO HEART

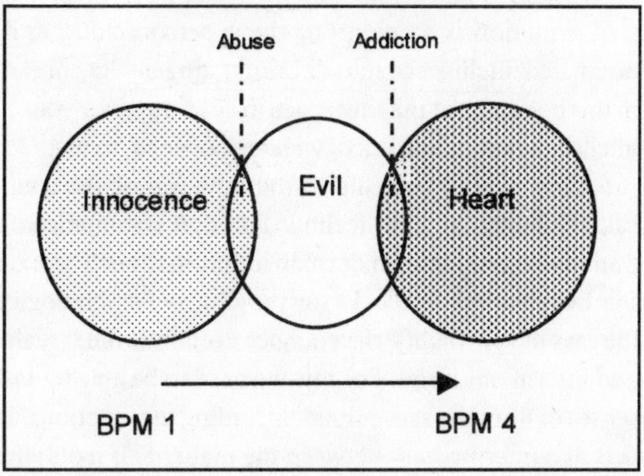

My model sees evil as a *necessary evil*, which provides us with the opportunities to develop and strengthen our will.

Life without will is impossible. Every thought, every movement requires us to use our will. But it is a different story to align our will to the Divine Will (God's Will). The journey from innocence to heart is about that alignment. It is about learning; it is about gaining the wisdom that is necessary to move inside and beyond.

> Divine Will has no boundaries; it works through laws known and unknown, natural and seemingly miraculous. It can change the course of destiny, wake the dead, cast mountains into the sea, and create new solar systems.
>
> Man, as an image of God, possesses within him that all-accomplishing power of will. To discover through right meditation how to be in harmony with the Divine Will is man's highest obligation.
>
> When guided by error, human will misleads us; but when guided by wisdom, human will is attuned to the Divine Will. God's plan for us often becomes obscured by the conflicts of human life and so we lose the inner guidance that would save us from chasms of misery.[62]

The greenhouse situation certainly makes sure that we lose our inner guidance and use instead the outer guidance of consumerism, greed and envy. Strong will is a requirement in industry and commerce. But what is favoured is a ruthless will that is not connected with the heart. It is a will that is connected with many of the evil qualities above, a will that usually lingers in the shadowy areas of abuse and addiction.

Wisdom

What then is this wisdom that we need to gain on the journey through the darkness from innocence to heart, in order to come out the other side with a strong will that is attuned to Divine Will?

Wisdom is knowledge and intuition, or intellect guided by the intuition of the soul. Intuition is a quality of the superconscious, and turns ordinary externally orientated intelligence into discriminating intelligence. All the chapters and models in this book aim at making space in your mind for your intuition and wisdom. Your intellect is being sharpened, widened, opened, to include mental models (maps) that can allow you to open up to the intuition of the soul. Undeveloped intuition is called a hunch or a gut feeling. Through systematic yoga meditation and concentration exercises we can develop intuition to such an extent that it leads to wisdom. It is like clearing the blocks surrounding the psychological greenhouse space so that the rays of spirituality, the energies from the higher realms can come through again and inform our mind. For this we need to be able to withdraw life energy from the senses or from the sense-mind, including the emotions. But it is our intelligence that acts as a intermediary between the higher Self (soul) and the sense-mind.

Consciousness (Chitta) is closer to the Self while the sense-mind (Manas) is closer to the ego. Intelligence (Buddhi), which is placed between them, is the key factor in how we orientate our awareness. Because of its capacity for decisive perception, intelligence has the power of spiritual transformation greater than either the sense-mind or deeper consciousness. It can empty consciousness of its conditioning and control the sense-mind. It can question the ego and discriminate between the lower and the higher Self.[63]

It is interesting to note here that in Vedic psychology, intelligence is not at all a bad thing. Rational intelligence is not dismissed in favour of the emotions as is popular with many trendy pseudo-psychology approaches. On the contrary, emotions are seen as part of the sense-mind, expressing likes and dislikes, attraction and repulsion in relation to the objects of the senses including thoughts. Part of the journey is therefore to withdraw energy from the emotions as part of the senses. But Vedic psychology does differentiate between outer intelligence and inner intelligence. Outer intelligence is wholly informed by the outer world through the sense-mind, while inner or higher intelligence is informed through the soul.

I should like to think that the maps and models in this book contribute to you, the reader, learning to see things differently, thus de-conditioning your consciousness and developing your higher intelligence or wisdom.

When all the senses are stilled, when the mind is at rest, when the intellect wavers not – that, say the wise, is the highest state. This calm of the senses and the mind has been defined as yoga. He who attains it is freed from delusion.[64]

9

Senseless Senses

The energy that charges our senses comes from cosmic life energy and enters our body through the *medulla oblongata*, a point at the back of the head where the spine enters the skull. The life energy then goes out from the head through the different chakras (energy centres) along the spine, and from there into our senses, organs, limbs. The aim in meditation is to draw this energy back into the brain and the spine. Soul is the experience of life energy being centred in brain and spine. There are also a wide range of healing techniques, including cranial osteopathy that deal with blocks of the energy flow along the spine and the chakras ('opening the chakras').

According to Vedic wisdom it is mainly cosmic life energy that keeps us alive. In our bodies that life energy is mainly pulled into the senses. Note! Life energy is pulled out into the senses, and meditation is then about reversing that process. Yogananda often uses the image of a camera for the sense of sight. He says that the mind uses life energy to photograph objects through the eye. Potentially we could use our eyes to see far more than they actually do; for example, we could have X-ray vision. But through convention and conditioning, we have limited what we see.

Another way of understanding this rather different way of understanding would be to ponder that a dead person cannot see. But when alive, our senses are charged with life energy and we can see, hear, touch, smell. Similarly, no matter how much food you stuff into a dead person, she will not live.

We can see how in the greenhouse world most of the life energy is constantly pulled out through the senses by objects of desire, thus distancing us from soul. In its extreme forms these sense attachments turn into addictions. Let us explore addictions as extreme expressions of sense attachments.

Sex can be bad for you

Robert had done a lot of work to come through his depression, which was mainly caused by stress at work and by problems in his relationship with Stephen. Robert had a very cynical attitude towards the promiscuity of many of their homosexual friends. He did not like Stephen's rather relaxed approach to sex. Robert felt that his and Stephen's views about

life and their future were drifting apart. Then, one day, he decided to have sex with a much
younger man who was visiting him and Stephen. Even though he did not feel it was a 'big
deal', he started to fantasise about that young man, and for the first time ever he began to
have sexual interactions in gay chat rooms on the internet.

Robert's example shows how easily sex can serve as a distraction; how it can
be used as a weapon; how it can push us to act against our better knowledge or
our values; and how it can lead to addictive behaviour. Let us now explore sex as
the most powerful activity of the sense-mind.

Sex involves the most intense energisation of the senses of smelling, hearing,
seeing, touching and tasting. In sexual arousal life energy is drawn into the senses
to a degree that would otherwise only be possible in the fight-flight reaction to life-
threatening situations. To be highly 'sensed up' also means to be highly prone to
conditioning, i.e. powerful sense memories are created in the mind, and, in the
case of pleasant memories a craving for the repetition of the experience becomes
firmly installed. In the case of highly charged unpleasant sense experiences, the
avoidance of similar situations can become an obsession, leading to, or strengthening conditions like anxiety disorders, depression, obsessive compulsive
disorder.[65]

In our culture the strong repetition urge that is created by the sexual charging
of the senses is generally regarded as positive, while the anxiety related charging
of the senses is regarded as neurotic and requiring therapy. Sexuality and the associated repetition urge are generally regarded as a good thing, despite the fact that
it can lead to obsessions and addictions because of its sense-nature. Because of
its potential to lead to easy conditioning (habit forming) sexuality is increasingly
used to promote and sell all sorts of things. Similarly, at the opposite end of the
spectrum, the absence of fear and threat is also being used to promote products,
lifestyles and services.

We can now see how all the maps we have developed and the dynamics we have
explored so far are essentially based in this core process of drawing life energy out
into the senses, and in the associated habit of the mind to store sense memories as
action plans for either repetition or avoidance. This is how the world of matter and
senses works. It is based on drawing life energy out – expansion (into the senses
in our example). The opposite movement is pulling in or contraction. In Vedic
cosmology it is the interplay between expansion and contraction that created and
is creating the universe. Contraction, e.g. the pulling back of sense energy or the
formation of black holes, is seen by the rishis as the way back to God. The only
way out is in. The most powerful sense attachments are related to sexuality and to
fear (of death). They are absolutely vital for survival as long as we think that this
life in the world of matter is all there is. Our lack of spirituality (see greenhouse
model) has consequently blown sex and pleasure addiction and fear-related avoidance out of all proportion. And as long as we do not believe in eternal soul and
spirit we cannot but go on further into addictions and fear.

HUNGRY BABIES

At this point I should like to include my thoughts about writing about sexuality. I am worried, and I need to ask myself why I am worried. I am worried about your, the reader's, possibly negative reactions to what I am writing. It is a very touchy subject to write about, especially as my basic premise is that sex can be not good for you, and can even be hazardous to your mental and spiritual health. How can someone like me who grew up in the 1960s, and lived through the 'sexual liberation' of the 1970s come up with prudish stuff like this? Don't we all know with deep certainty that sex is good for us? We are being told that repressed sexuality can lead to all manner of emotional drama. We are supposed to have a fulfilled sex life, and if we don't, we had better go and see a sex therapist. It's the peak of intimacy. It's 'making love'. It releases stress and tension. And, above all, it makes us feel good. And feeling good is good, isn't it?

I think that my concern about your reaction to what I am trying to put across, may in itself say something about how uncritically we all (including me) accept our attachment to sense-gratification. It is very difficult to look and think beyond. Repressed sexuality brings up images of priests abusing young boys, monks raping young girls. So we want to be liberal and have a healthy sex life. We may even see sexual ecstasy as the way to spiritual fulfilment. The freedom to follow the call of sense pleasures has become our god. I think we need to re-think and put sexuality into a proper spiritual context, which, for me, means to fully acknowledge and process the dangers that seem quite obviously implicit in the apple.

Perhaps we can understand and accept it better when we use a psychological map to look at sexuality, because psychological models are more easily acceptable to the sense-identified intellect or mind.

Men especially often get worried when they are not in a relationship with a woman. 'Holding it all in' seems wrong. Life without sex feels like a slippery slope into death.

> It was the Victorians who repressed sexuality, but today we are obsessed with sexuality and repress death. Sex is used defensively and almost compulsively as proof against ageing and death.[66]

In our culture sex is equated with vitality, strength, alive-ness. Sex serves as the repeated confirmation that life is 'eternal', and that total merger with another person, with something beyond our limited personal self, is possible. In a sense sex carries many spiritual connotations. What we are less aware of is that it can also be the futile attempt to recapture the intimacy the infant did not have with his mother. Rich material for many years of psychotherapy – but no resolution in sight. Of course, the psycho-dynamics of sex are very relevant, but only if we see them in a spiritual context.

Without going too much into the complexities of psychoanalytical models, we can easily imagine how important the very early bonding between mother and baby is. This is the arena where the baby learns about relationships, intimacy, and above all, what it means to be himself. We can also imagine how difficult all this can be. Mothers are often unprepared and overwhelmed by this totally dependent creature. They can feel as if they have to sacrifice their 'self' in order to give it to the baby. Resentment, ambivalence, over-protectiveness can so easily come into this early relationship. Mistakes occur. No-one is to blame – really. But often the babies spend the rest of their lives trying to make up for the shortcomings of those vital early weeks, months, years.

Relationships and especially sex can then be the arena where the adult tries to work out his or her baby stuff. It can all become very confusing for everyone concerned. The former babies keep looking for fulfilment and bliss in their adult relationships, but never find it. Their partners may be on a similar search, or may become bewildered by the other's insatiable needs, their ambivalence, their infidelity. The relationship drama is in full flow. New babies are born into old unresolved dramas and new grown-up 'hungry babies' are created.

We now seem to be living in a world full of grown-up hungry babies. And in a way it is not that important when it all started. It is here with us now, and sex and consumerism have become an integral part of it, because hungry babies crave intimacy and they want to be fed, especially with sex.

So now we have this unholy alliance – hungry babies and a world economy that relies on hungry customers. The advertising industry, powerful and rich enough to use the world's top intelligence and creativity, has the task to identify and use the hunger, maintain it, and create more hunger. They are doing it well. And they do it in a brilliantly hidden manner. Their activities enter our hungry baby unconscious need patterns through skilfully worded, displayed and presented commercial messages everywhere. But at the same time their activities enter our rational adult minds only as economic data, turnover, profits, share prices and return on investment. This is a brilliant system. Nothing is what it seems. Is it paranoid to assume that, maybe, just maybe, this system may also have a vested interest in making sure that hungry babies are created from the very start?

Sex has become the focus for all those unfulfilled needs for intimacy. It is the focus because it carries so much sense-energy, the need for repetition and the potential for permanent hunger. Sex is used in advertising to sell goods, services and lifestyles. We know that somewhere deep down, but we still fall for it. What I am suggesting here is that the 'system' may also have an interest in creating the conditions where sex can be used, and continue to be used as the 'big pull'.

If you were the big controller, who can see all the connections, how then would you go about making sure that there is a constant flow of hungry babies? Obviously, you would try and create mothering and fathering conditions that set the scene, that create the 'material' you can use. What conditions would you want?

Single mothers – yes.
Disintegrating marriages – yes.
Stressed, poor, unemployed parents – yes.
Survival fears – yes.
Lack of social support – yes.
Unprepared parents – yes.

Sexual temptations for both men and women all over the place are ideal to achieve the above conditions. And it is also ideal to tease the hungry babies, and to keep them hungry and craving for the rest of their lives. In contrast, just imagine what it would be like if we did not have hungry babies.

This could all sound like a conspiracy theory. That someone, somewhere is scheming to create those conditions. Some people might think that it is the devil, some dark power or dark forces, or even groups of people creating those conditions. I prefer the Hindu concept of maya to understand it. Everything in the universe is connected; the same patterns are everywhere. The focus of our explorations has been how the process of splitting and fragmentation operates on different psychological and societal levels and how we are all caught up in it like in a web or a maze. Many personal development approaches aim at freeing sexuality from all its neurotic and destructive connotations. They want people to get back to the *pure* sexuality that to them represents passion, freedom, liberation, spirit. Those schools of thought would, no doubt, join me in my outrage about the abusive sexuality that is surrounding us in our culture. But they do believe that sexual energy is just perverted by capitalism, consumerism etc., and that, once freed from those powers, it can again be what is was meant to be – pure love and joy of the soul.

I think it is far more complicated than this. It is not just the inadequate or neurotic sexual development of individuals that needs to be addressed here, but a sexual confusion that runs all the way through our culture. Sex has become the energetic glue for the splitting, fragmentation and sense-orientation that surrounds and pervades us. And, as we have discussed, sexuality offers itself for this role because of its strong sense-connections, and because of its potential to maintain hungry babies.

It may help us here to use the model of the journey from innocence to heart (see Fig. 7 on p. 105). We can see how the innocent sexuality of the child needs to move on to an adult sexuality that is contained by the heart. However, in our culture sexual development seems to have become arrested in the middle section of the chart labelled *evil* (or somewhere between BPM 2 and BPM 3). Rather than moving on to heart, sexuality then circles around in the middle section of evil, and can move on to a pseudo-heart position, or it moves back to a pseudo-innocence. These are the overlap areas in the chart, where abuse can be seen as an attempt to re-capture innocence by using power, and where addictive sexuality can be seen as the futile attempt to achieve union through compulsion without first addressing the fragmented character of sexuality, thus further solidifying the fragmentation.

Even the yogic world seems to be split when it comes to sexuality. There are those, who, on the basis of seeing sexuality as one of the most powerful forces of duality and delusion, advocate either celibacy or its sole use in the process of procreation. And then there are some tantric schools who use sexual techniques as a force for transformation. I think there are dangers with both extremes. The former school can easily lead to a puritan, punitive, and guilt-ridden attitude towards sex. The tantric side carries the danger of ignoring the destructive potential of sexuality that we have been exploring here.

It will not be possible to resolve these issues in this book. But perhaps the model of the chakras can give us some further clues. Spiritual development is seen as the movement of energy up the spine – from the lower centres to the higher ones. The heart centre is in the middle position between the higher and lower centres. In a way it holds the balance between the two. Fragmented and destructive sexuality pulls the energy down into the lower centres of solar plexus, sacrum and base of spine, thus creating a counter-movement to the energetic upward journey of the spiritual path. Hence there needs to be a strong connection between sexuality and heart, or, sexual energy needs to be held by the heart. It is the heart that can ensure that spiritual advancement and sexuality can be balanced and maybe even complement each other.

Addictions are in the Mind

Peter has done a lot of work on his depression which was caused by his girlfriend leaving him just before they were supposed to get married. A few months beforehand Peter had started to have sex with prostitutes. The girlfriend did not know about this. Now, many years and a girlfriend later he is still having sex with prostitutes. Usually he books them through an agency to visit him at home. Afterwards he always feels ashamed and very determined never to do it again. But within a few weeks the excitement usually builds up again. He, again, goes through his elaborate ritual of making telephone contact with the agency, choosing a particular girl, making sure his car is parked away from his house in case his girlfriend might visit unexpectedly. The thought that one more time would not matter, and that he would definitely stop it after this time, is always running in the back of his mind. This is now making him depressed. He has also started to use pornographic internet sites in an addictive manner.

Earlier I mentioned how important it is to talk to the rational mind in order to allow the intuitive mind some space. Well, that's not the whole story. The rational mind also needs to be questioned and disciplined. But it does not need to be disciplined by telling it to 'become more emotional'. It needs to be disciplined with regard to what it should be rational about. For example, your rational mind might consider it perfectly ok for you to drink a bottle of whisky every Saturday, especially because you usually drink only five pints of beer per night during the rest of the week. After all, you feel good when you have a drink at the end of a hard working day, and weekends are for relaxing anyway. 'It's all about feeling good', your rational mind says, and you are convinced that life is about feeling good. Let's explore what 'feeling good' means in this instance. Your mind is telling you that it feels good when it experiences a different range of sensations as a result of the amount of alcohol in you. Your mind defines 'feeling good' in a sense-focused way. It is quite clear that in this example you would need to discipline your mind. But how would you do it? I can think of many patients who were quite clearly drinking far too much far too regularly. But often they could not see any reason for stopping, and just discipline would not work then. So your mind needs different models, different maps in order for any discipline to work. I strongly believe that those maps have to be about spirituality. Remember, the only way out is in. So, let's see how we can explain to the rational mind that it is very easy to get caught up in the 'feeling good' loop in a world where attachments and addictions are the norm. But we also want to put across to the rational mind that this norm is only a made-up one, and not the whole reality.

Desires are habits of the senses and they manifest at the level of the mind and ideas.

> It is when the mind becomes attached to a sensation that it develops a correspondingly pleasing idea in the brain. This pleasant idea about a sensation causes an individual to repeat his experiences with that sensation. When a sensation is constantly repeated, it causes a repetition of its corresponding pleasing idea in the brain. This liking idea becomes 'grooved' in the brain and fixed in the mind as a mental habit. This mental habit – formed by repeating a pleasing idea that evolved from a sensation – is what causes the attractiveness of sensations. Just as everybody is more or less in love with his own ideas about things, whether they are right or not, so also, the mind likes his own personal collection of mental sense habits. [A pleasing sensation] is [nothing but] an idea liked by another idea.[67]

Ideas that are liked by ideas that are liked by ideas that are liked by ideas – and on it goes. It becomes easy to imagine what the psychological greenhouse looks like inside our heads. Once sequences and circles of ideas are created and solidified into habits, new pleasure-seeking ideas and actions can expand the sequences into complex systems of a pseudo-reality. Fragments of sensations and memories that are connected in our minds through pleasing ideas about sensations and activities that are based on those ideas, only to form more ideas, more activities to repeat the sensations. We are driven by a lethal combination of sensations and thoughts about those sensations.

This system includes our conscious and unconscious memories in the following way. The mind has a sense-pleasing memory and the mind likes that sense-pleasing memory. It then wants to re-create the sense situation that created the memory in the first place. Hence action is being taken to re-create that situation, or mental pattern. The more unclear or vague the memory is, the more different from the original the desired situation or mental pattern can be and still satisfy the mind's craving. That is why deeply unconscious memories can create a striving for sense constellations that are quite different from the original constellation that created the memory in the first place. We can even apply this to deeply buried, hardly conscious past-life memories. Then, once the sense constellation has been re-created, a new memory is being formed that strengthens the initial memory (this is similar to Grof's COEX model – see p. 60). Here we need to take into account the holographic character of memory. The memory constellation covers the whole brain and creates a reality that becomes stronger every time it is reinforced. It even connects with other aspects within the whole hologram – other people's stuff, collective stuff, etc.

This is why 'withdrawing life energy from the senses', including sense-memories, is such a vital thing, because it cuts into this repetitive process of mind – memory – liking memory – re-creating sense constellation – reinforcing holographic memory – reinforcing reality. And it cuts in at the only place where the cycle can be interrupted. We cannot change memories, but we can stop reinforcing them and we can stop creating new ones. We can stop allowing the COEX from the past to create the reality for the future. And we do that by cutting the reinforcing process in the present.

This is the why meditation and withdrawing energy from the senses is so important. It is not just some kind of abstract renunciation, but it is about creating a future that is not totally determined by the past (the conscious and unconscious past).

But then the psychological greenhouse system tells us to do exactly the opposite. Advertising is specifically aimed at stimulating deep semi-conscious and unconscious sense memories and even soul memories are turned into sense memories to dominate our actions. And apart from the specifics we also *learn the process itself*. We are trained to trust pleasing sense memories and to constantly reinforce them.

The One More Time Syndrome

Then when we have decided to let go of an old destructive habit, the mind says: *Just one more go; just one more beer; just one more binge; just one more wild night out; just one more time with this or that favourite fantasy. Discipline can start tomorrow.*

This *just one more time and then we'll stop* is the seductive voice of the old sense-habits defending their position or trying to find their way back in. *From tomorrow you will lead a different life; so today doesn't really matter, today doesn't really count.* It is the way in which the voice of the senses uses the finality of life to trick us back into our old ways. If we believe that this life is all we have, then the thought of never again doing or feeling this or that pleasing thing, can be quite unbearable. We can become convinced that one more time really does not make that much difference. After all, the intention is the important thing, isn't it?

When we follow that voice, we unfortunately buy the whole package. It can become one more time until we die. We believe that as long as we can think and act from the position of one more time, we have a future. The moment gets stretched into a lifelong succession of one more times. Perfection, bliss is just around the corner. We can stop the old destructive ways at any moment, we believe.

At this stage we may well know intuitively that bliss will not be achieved through the senses, so we try to stretch out the letting go of sense addictions. One more for the road! And that makes it more intense. Each 'one more time' giving-in becomes more intense and leaves a bigger imprint. Then the next stage is when we notice how our newly developed discipline and soul-qualities are drifting away. They become a faint memory. *I can't do it anyway; might as well give up and give in.* The senses are winning. *Maybe this is how far I can go in this life* – resignation and accepting that this is how life is. By then *one more time* has turned into *it doesn't matter anyway*. The path is lost again and we are wading in the sticky mud of the slough of despond once more.

Or you might go and do some 'reality testing' which can be extremely confusing, because 'reality' confirms the 'one more time' and 'doesn't matter anyway' attitudes that have settled in your mind. You look around you and you see sexual and other sense stimuli everywhere. Women and especially young girls in sexy clothes are freely splashed on billboards, packaging, cinema and TV programmes. Pick up a few hundred pages of explicit and 'exciting' pornography in WH Smith's (sold as women writing for women even though a man writes it, and probably mostly men read it). Find yourself a woman in her twenties from Asia or Russia to 'buy' on the Internet or some other sense (sex) stimulation. So there, that is the world we live in, so it must be normal. It's reality.

There you are. Reality seems to be mainly about stimulating your senses, preferably all of them at once. The big 'come-on' is surrounding you. And it is all seriously and genuinely very tempting and exciting, all strengthening the 'one more time' and 'doesn't matter anyway' attitude. Be 'real' – join in and remain hungry again and again and again and again until you die. Perhaps old age will give you some relief, when the senses begin to close down for death. You can then be a 'wise old person'. It seems to be the only area where our culture accepts wisdom. But then, old age is looked down upon, pitied, in the world of the senses.

So there you are with your strengthened and reality-confirmed attitudes of 'one more time' and 'doesn't matter anyway'. What do you then do with the faint glimpses of NO that still pop up in your mind at times? The vague memories of past New Year's resolutions, of the guilt-driven resolve after the last painful disaster. It's easy to let go of them, isn't it, because it is all so exciting.

But can you see how close the 'one-more-time-doesn't-matter-anyway' attitude is to depression? Can it ultimately lead to anything but depression? Take pubs, for example. There are the exciting flirtatious ones, full of young people carrying out their mating rituals. And then there are the really depressed ones, the 'drinking holes', for the middle or even old-aged men and women who spend their time topping up the accumulated alcohol levels of wasted decades. Excitement is for youth, depression is for old age, alcohol and sex (or the lack of it) are for both, and lead the way from one to the other. In youth alcohol mainly serves to stimulate excitement, to loosen inhibitions. Later on in life it serves to dampen the depression. And, of course, there is the physical addiction. What can you do after a period of heavy sense stimulation other than withdraw, get depressed?

Alcohol and sex have served here as examples for illustrating sense attachments and addictions, and how those attachments are woven into the greenhouse system. Other sense attachments like over-eating, shopping and gambling follow similar patterns. You will also, hopefully, have realised how the normal mind is intimately connected with the senses and keeps the attachments going mainly through sense-memories and through the resultant urge for repetition of those pleasurable experiences. Even when we think that we have overcome a certain attachment or addiction, the *army* of the senses often re-groups and fights back like in the *one more time syndrome*. This battle is powerfully described in the *Bhagavad Gita*.

The Pub

The beast is like a breast,
a good breast,
or so it seems.

Beer flows freely,
blurring the brain
and every cell of the body.

The breast we never had,
or were afraid of.
Now we're bonding with the taps,
through the barmaids.

Cricket on the green,
the statue of a lion,
proudly towers in a dark corner.

Conversation is low tonight,
in the pub.

The beer flows freely,
filling the fault inside
with liquid and with alcohol.
The liquid disappears slowly
in the sand
at the bottom of the fault.

The alcohol stays a bit longer,
lulling the senses,
so the gap doesn't seem
quite so deep,
quite so dark,
for a while.

But alcohol eats away
at the solid edges of the gap,
widening it,
deepening it,

more sand at the bottom,
a bigger gap to fill.

The conversation is picking up now,
bar talk,
roaring laughter.
Words spoken and not recalled,
words heard and not remembered.

Bar talk, pub talk.
The world is put right here,
with no effect whatsoever.
Words disappear,
like the liquid in the sand
at the bottom of the fault,
leaving the hangover of unfulfilled dreams,
of un-remembered connections,
in the dream-world of the pub.

A feeling of something new,
of future,
when the pint glass is still fairly full.
Then the death at the bottom of the glass,
when the last bit of beer
has gone stale and warm.

But the barmaid still handles the breast,
the tap pours another pint
of amber liquid,
into the transparent container.

Jokes are entering the conversation now,
men roar, women too,
fun, enjoyment, fun.

The clock ticks away,
counting time,
counting life,
in the dream of the safe womb,
the womb that even has a breast.

Now the pub is shut.

The breast dried out.
No home to go to,
no safe space
protected by ancient wooden beams,
by alcoholic liquid.

No friends any more,
friends who were searching for the same
unspoken, but communicated,
unheard, but felt
desire for a safe home,
where you can come and go as you please,
accepted and always welcome.
Where they know your name.

Gone, the stillness where time stood still,
for a moment,
for a few hours,
for a few pints,
for a few people.
The longing continues as a craving.

10

Maps for the Soul

It is all pretty gruesome – splitting, fragmentation, consumerism, greed, envy, psychological greenhouse, addictions. Can this really be the world we live in and carry around inside us? Isn't this just a one-sided analysis that completely ignores the many elements of bliss and happiness that are also part of our lives? Is it just that I, as a psychotherapist, am biased towards the dark, suffering side of life and humanity?

The models and maps that we have developed so far in this book do not differentiate between inner and outer worlds. They present a holographic view of the universe and ourselves: we are an integral part of everything else and everything else is an integral part of us. This is also what I experience with my clients. They present to me their individual expression of much larger issues and problems; and I can see and feel the larger whole through them. Their individual condition is only an expression of the larger human condition.

How can I not see a connection between someone with depression and the fact that the prescription rate for antidepressants has been increasing enormously in recent years, and that suicides amongst young men are going up rapidly? How can I ignore the connection between an individual's violent rage and the caged lifestyles (greenhouse) that most people are forced to lead? How can I not see a connection between eating disorders and how I sometimes want to scream in the supermarket that I do not want to have to choose between ten different brands and sizes of baked beans or bread? How can I not feel compassion for men who become addicted to pornography or telephone sex, when their sex drive is being stimulated every day in order to sell cars, computers, mobile phones, beer, chewing gum, coffee – to name just a few? How can I not feel hopelessness and helplessness as a psychotherapist when my clients drag the bits of the global drama that they carry, into my consulting room? Can I then say to them that it can be fixed because I know someone or they know someone who is happy, successful in this world or despite this world?

No, the *fixing it* within the drama seems too superficial a way. It goes against the holistic view that we have been developing on these pages. But I can help my clients to see themselves, that is, their interdependent inner and outer worlds, more clearly, and I can help them to go to a different place inside themselves where they can feel peace and calm and even bliss (not as an escape!), and from where they can project a different energy into the whole web-like hologram. Yogananda writes:

> Find joy within and express it in your face. When you do that, wherever you go a little smile will surcharge everyone with your divine magnetism. Everybody will be happy![68]

But this projection of energy out from that deep place of peace and calm, in other words from the soul, has a bigger effect than just magnetising others and making them happy. It puts a positive piece into the collective soup, into that hologram of thoughts and feelings that surrounds and permeates all of us. By going inside and projecting energy out from our soul we are influencing other people and the world around us in direct *and* in more subtle, indirect ways. Examples to illustrate the latter would be processes where the action of the mind has an effect on others' minds and on matter, like telepathy, telekinesis, or healing. In his book *The Holographic Universe*, Michael Talbot gives many well researched examples and case studies of 'miraculous' events, and he quotes well known scientists expressing their beliefs:

> In private conversation Bohm admits to believing that the universe is all 'thought' and reality only exists in what we think ... . Pribram is similarly reticent to comment on specific events but does believe a number of different potential realities exist and consciousness has a certain amount of latitude in choosing which one manifests. ... Watson is bolder: 'I have no doubt that reality is in a very large part a construct of the imagination. I am not speaking as a particle physicist or even as someone who is totally aware of what's going on in the frontier of that discipline, but I think we have the capacity to change the world around us in quite fundamental ways'.[69]

So we can make our contribution to changing the world by switching off the senses and going inside ourselves. We have to do this by going to the stillness beyond the sense and thought-orientated mind.

> Only if we change our deepest thoughts can we really change ourselves and get beyond the limitations of the mind. This is much more than changing our ideas about things; it means altering our deepest feelings and instincts. It requires deep prayer and meditation, profoundly energized and concentrated higher thought forms to counter deep-seated habits and addictions.[70]

By going beyond the mind to that deep place called soul or inner Self or higher Self, we will find peace and relaxation for ourselves, and we will also be doing important work for a better world. Let's try a story.

THE REVOLUTIONARY AND THE YOGI (REFLECTION 8)

The revolutionary is worn out from all his fighting for a better world. His body and mind are exhausted from his battles – some won, some lost. He did achieve some important changes for the people of his country. The cruel dictator eventually had to flee, but he managed to take all his wealth with him. Now there is an elected democratic government in place, but there is still corruption, and some of the new politicians are forgetting how hard the revolutionary had to fight and risk his life countless times to get them into their places of power. The revolutionary has become bitter, cynical and he is disappointed with what he now calls 'human nature'. And then there was the earthquake. So many people got killed, and many tried to take advantage from the chaos and the shortages – looting, murders, corruption. The decent people that were left were crying out for a strong leader again, and they started to blame the revolutionary for their misery. They even wanted the old dictator back. The revolutionary is fed up with revolution and he takes his worn out and wounded body into the mountains. After a long and strenuous journey he comes to a cave, in front of which sits a yogi deep in meditation. The yogi looks so peaceful and still – even from a distance the revolutionary can feel the energy from the meditating yogi reach right to his heart. The revolutionary breaks down in front of the yogi and cries and cries until he has no more tears left. With a broken voice he asks the yogi: 'What have I done wrong?' The yogi smiles and replies …

What do you think the yogi replied?

What was your very first thought about how you wanted to complete the story?

What thoughts and feelings were stirred up in you while you read the story?

Spend a few moments reflecting on the three questions.

The story is meant to stimulate your intuition and your wisdom. You will probably have identified with the revolutionary's struggles and disappointments. You will by now, hopefully, have a sense of wanting to do it differently. The yogi represents your own inner voice of wisdom – the voice that comes out of the intuition of your soul. How does what you wanted the yogi to reply relate to your past and present struggles?

My point is, that the important work we need to do is inner work first and then outer work. By being examples, whether we are politicians, managers, secretaries, housewives or carpenters, we can have an effect on the people we come in contact with. And we can create an energy field that surrounds us and goes beyond us. By changing our own self we are changing the universe, because each one of us is a unique and central part of the universe, of creation. By changing one part, the whole cannot remain the same. We are co-creators in more ways than one.

Gandhi was someone who tried to achieve a balance between inner and outer work. He had clear political and economic goals and he gave his life for those goals. He used himself as an example of simplicity, and non-violence as the weapon of resistance. He resisted evil by the force of love.

Politics as spiritualized by Gandhi, and the consecrated altars of the hearts of men God-illumined through meditation, can establish the heaven of peace within and without in the family, social, political, and spiritual life of men.[71]

And, in Gandhi's own words:

Always aim at complete harmony of thought and word and deed. Always aim at purifying your thoughts and everything will be well. There is nothing more potent than thought. Deed follows word and word follows thought. The world is the result of a mighty thought and where the thought is mighty and pure the result is always mighty and pure.[72]

So how do we get to this inner place of peace and calm, to that place of stillness, to our soul? First of all we obviously need to withdraw our energy from the greenhouse space that is surrounding us. Let us reflect for a moment on what you may have discovered so far about your way of life and about the way your mind arranges your life.

YOUR LIFE PATTERN (REFLECTION 9)

You should by now have recognised:–
your own ways of splitting and fragmentation,
the alienation in your life,
your own inner greenhouse,
the way in which your mind reacts to a different way of seeing things,
your addictions and attachments,
the way in which your mind tries to hold on to old habits.

You may even have some ideas about the pattern of your life. These are issues, struggles, disappointments, problems that arise throughout your life in the same or in a similar way. There usually is a pattern that runs through everybody's life. It usually is this pattern that keeps us stuck and prevents us from moving on. The pattern is your lesson, the dark forest on your hero's quest.

See if you can be quite specific about your pattern, rather than just naming it after the strong emotions that it repeatedly creates, e.g. anxiety, depression, anger, etc. The emotional labels for your pattern will not help you to change anything. They tend to be regarded as symptoms that require treatment with medication. If you, however, specify your pattern using the psycho-spiritual maps and models from this book, you will arrive at a formulation that goes beyond emotional suffering and that will allow you to go beyond the mind. Thus you will begin to hand over control of your life to the soul.

As much as you can, do an honest life evaluation. Use the material from all the previous reflections in this book, especially your greenhouse map and the greenhouse qualities that are relevant for you for your evaluation.

The Three-Dimensional Egg

We are now trying to develop maps for the journey beyond the mind, the journey to the soul. How can you leave the old habits, the old ways of thinking behind? If you have read and reflected thus far, your mind has somehow been dealing with the material you have been reading, and you will have already begun to clear the path inside. You have taken the first steps on the path. Your mind will have also, no doubt, been trying to block, reject, forget anything that felt too threatening to its old established ways. It would still be very easy to just go back and regard it all as an interesting, intellectually stimulating exercise. But we cannot leave it just at the level of intellectual stimulation if we want to go on a spiritual path. That level of fascination and interest might occasionally blow your mind, but it does not go beyond the mind. In order to go beyond the mind we need to do more.

I am now trying to make the case for meditation, the case for yoga more directly. 'The only way out is in' implies that there is no other way out of the greenhouse. Otherwise I would have chosen a title like 'one of the ways out is in'. But the title specifically states that we do not have a choice here. We shall now be exploring exactly why this is so and what that means.

A new map will help us understand what we have been doing and where we are going. The model is an expansion of the egg diagram in the chapter on the psychological greenhouse.

I find Assagioli's original egg quite either-or, in that it separates the higher from the lower unconscious in a rather drastic way. You can either go up into the higher unconscious or down into the lower half. Or, the journey to the higher Self (the star) can, more realistically, be seen as a spiral (see Fig. 8). Whenever we move up into the higher realms, we soon dig up some complex or issue from the lower unconscious. An example would be that when we have decided to be more compassionate towards our fellow human beings, someone plays a really nasty trick on us. We feel cheated, angry, enraged. We want revenge, because the situation is similar to how we felt cheated as a child, when 'being good' did not get us anywhere. In this example the intention from the higher realms has stirred up a longstanding conflict from the lower unconscious. And so the journey goes on – up and down like a roller-coaster.

Psychosynthesis therapy, for example, can be defined as trying to offer its clients the guidance and 'working through' that is needed on this spiral-shaped journey. It is the role of the therapist to help the client face and resolve blocks and issues from the lower unconscious, while at the same time never losing sight of the fact that the client's soul wants Self-realisation, i.e. that the client is trying to reach, or re-connect with, their higher Self.

The deliberations about Richard's striving for perfection in Chapter 3 would be a good example for a psychosynthesis approach to a client's problems. Reflections 8 and 9 above would also be examples. They aim at stimulating you

FIG. 8: THE PSYCHO-SPIRITUAL PROCESS

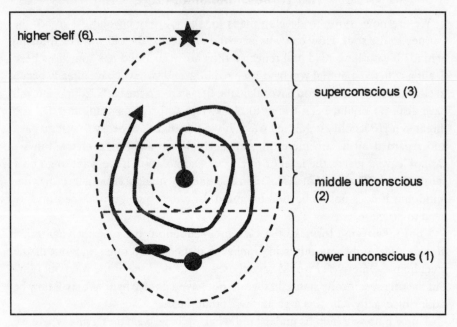

to listen to your inner voice, and at helping you understand your life pattern. All this is, obviously, good stuff. Spiritually, it goes beyond most other psychotherapy approaches. Why then, you may quite rightly ask, is going inside not the central part in psychosynthesis? Why do not all psychosynthesis therapists teach their clients meditation to withdraw life energy from the senses, and devotion to open the heart?

My criticism of the psychosynthesis model would be that it is only half a spiritual model. Very important things spiritual are missing. Yoga places a great deal of emphasis on spiritual values and practices that cover all important aspects of life. Many of the rules in yoga are there to contain and resolve the energies from the lower unconscious, so that they do not interfere with or pervert the spiritual development. The most important elements within the overall practice of right spiritual living are devotion and meditation. Neither are part of psychosynthesis, or of any other form of psychotherapy for that matter. But the absence of the core elements of spiritual practice are particularly damaging and dangerous in psychosynthesis, because it sees itself as a psycho-spiritual therapy and it does include spiritual elements in its thinking and its practice, like higher Self, the transpersonal, soul. It is then not surprising when the spiritual gaps in the model attract narcissistic ego qualities, or the ego grabs hold of it.

So, even though the psychosynthesis model can explain a lot about the ups and downs on our path, it cannot really explain why meditation and devotion have to be the central parts of the journey. Self-awareness and consciousness are central elements too, and they are vital, of course. But in the model as it stands, meditation is in danger of becoming just a technique to achieve or support that self-awareness. The spiral can easily turn into an endless going round in circles, because there is always more to be dug up in the lower unconscious; there is always more dark stuff that needs to be dragged to the light. I think that many people who spend many years in psychotherapy, including psychosynthesis, may have fallen into the trap of using meditation, going inside, purely as a therapeutic or self-development technique. This can then prevent them from proceeding on a proper spiritual path, which would have meditation and devotion as central elements.

It will help us move on to see the egg as a more circular, more ripple-like, and ultimately three-dimensional structure (see Fig. 9). Here the 'I', the centre of pure self-consciousness and the field of consciousness, are surrounded by the subconscious (called lower unconscious in the original egg), and this is then surrounded by the superconscious (called higher unconscious in the original egg). Seeing it like this feels more natural. It looks like ripples, the rings of tree trunks, atoms and neutrons, the solar system, waves, or the ripples on a holographic film.

The model in Fig. 9 also corresponds with the hierarchical order that Paramahansa Yogananda teaches in accordance with yogic science. The superconscious is the consciousness of the soul. When it descends into the brain and spine it becomes the subconscious; and when it goes into the nerves, muscles and senses it becomes consciousness. In this model the subconscious has the function of storing memories, but it also serves as a screen for its own and for superconscious images in dreams and dreamlike states. In yoga meditation it is important to learn to differentiate between subconscious and superconscious material. It is advisable to try and reduce purely subconscious images in dreams in order to make room for superconscious ones. The dark stuff that is stored in the subconscious mind is regarded pretty much as a nuisance that needs to be controlled and balanced with new good deeds and thoughts for healing to take place. This is, obviously, quite different from most Western psychotherapies, where the focus is very much on subconscious material to be worked through and resolved, which often takes many years. To summarise, I should like to quote Swami Akhilananda:

But a man need not be a mere creature of his past. The contents of the subconscious mind created by his own past thoughts and actions, as well as by the influence of others, can be changed or transformed

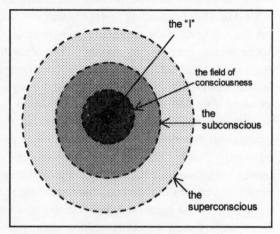

FIG. 9: THE PSYCHE AS RIPPLES

by the creating of new *samskaras*, or impressions. By changing the quality of his mental habits in the present, a man can himself direct and determine what his future mental state shall be. By regulating his thoughts and emotions, a man can make for himself new hope and new possibilities.[73]

I find this very refreshing, because it emphasises the importance of the here-and-now for the future. I wonder whether the emphasis on working on subconscious material that belongs to the past, found in most Western psychotherapy, could be another expression of the hungry baby syndrome that we explored earlier. Certainly, a powerful subconscious mind with lots of unresolved sense-cravings is vital for consumerism. At this point it might also be interesting to note that behaviour therapy and cognitive therapy, often dismissed as superficial, seem to approach therapy in a different and more Hindu way without, of course, having a spiritual perspective.

Seeing our psyche in this ripple format has implications for our considerations about the psychological greenhouse. Now there are no upper and lower parts in the diagram. Our field of consciousness would just be surrounded by objects from the subconscious, to some of which are glued elements from the superconscious. It is closing in on us from all sides, from all around us. And as in the earlier greenhouse model, the spiritual energies from the superconscious are blocked off.

But where is the higher Self here? Where is the star that was sitting on top of the egg in the earlier model, the place that we want to re-connect with? As the new ripple-model does not have an upper and lower part, only inner and outer, it seems difficult to place the higher Self anywhere. The only way we can now imagine it separate and central at the same time is to place the higher Self *beyond* the other levels of consciousness, which corresponds with the way it is described in yogic literature, as being beyond our three-dimensional world of matter and duality. This way of seeing it also resolves all the contentious issues around higher and lower. As we shall see, it also has practical implications for our journey inside.

I am therefore suggesting that the higher Self is situated in a dimension beyond – in the third one in the case of our two-dimensional ripples – and can therefore not be seen on the two-dimensional map. Rather than simply sitting on top of the egg, I suggest that the higher Self sits in a position that transcends the space of our two-dimensional map. Therefore, moving towards it becomes a process of transcending time and space as we normally know it. For example, if we take the two-dimensional ripples map as representing the ordinary three-dimensional space of our experience, then the higher Self can be found one dimension further on – in the fourth dimension, or in the third one on our map. This makes more sense to me than to just prop it on top of the egg, which, I think, positions it simply as part of the superconscious, thus not requiring any qualitative shift in being in order to reach it. I feel that this is where psychosynthesis has got it dangerously wrong, because it reduces the higher-dimension experience of self-realisation to a lower-dimensional practice that can be obtained through simple psychospiritual therapy, not requiring metaphysical practices and qualities like meditation and devotion.

Now, Fig. 10 has really exciting implications for us trying to get out of this greenhouse space. In the egg model we would have needed to break through the wall above in order to get through to the star at the top. But now this is turning into quite a different move.

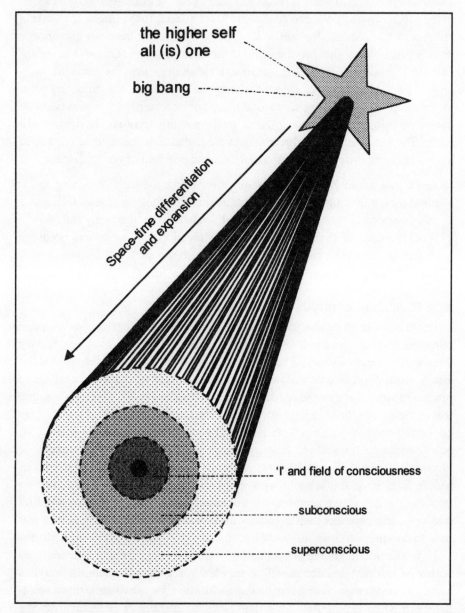

FIG. 10: THE THREE-DIMENSIONAL EGG

Look where the higher Self (= all is one = all-one = alone = God) is positioned in the three-dimension model. It is *behind* and *at the beginning/origin of* all our lower-dimensional levels of consciousness. It is apart and it is central. This is exciting! The higher Self is the point of origin, the big bang, of our conscious, subconscious and superconscious mind.[74] And this is where meditation and devotion are supposed to get us without us having to break through greenhouse walls, and without having to wade through the mud of the subconscious in order to get to the superconscious. We can go directly to the source, to the origin, the starting point of consciousness. But we do need to free ourselves from the greenhouse objects that hold us glued to the lower dimension (three-dimensional in reality, two-dimensional on map). Getting unstuck rather than breaking through!

And from which point do we get to the source? Not necessarily from any point in the subconscious or the superconscious, not necessarily from any point of deeply meaningful emotional suffering, or from highly spiritual mystical experiences. The easiest and most direct way to the higher Self seems to be from right here, from our centre of pure self-awareness and our field of consciousness.

> Right from this moment, bring discipline and watch the mind. Watching the mind means looking at your thoughts as they are, looking at your feelings and emotions as they are, without identifying them as 'this is my fear, this is my thought.' Without identification, justification, evaluation and notification, you can see a clear-cut gap between two thoughts, a space between two emotions. In that space there is a door. Enter into that door.[75]

THE CASE FOR SPIRITUAL PSYCHOTHERAPY

But in order to go on that journey to the higher Self we often need to 'un-glue' ourselves from all those greenhouse attachments that keep us stuck to ordinary three-dimensional existence. Fig. 9 on p. 127 and Fig. 11 on p. 131 show that the aim of meditation is to withdraw energy from the field of consciousness or the sense-mind into the 'I' or the centre of pure self-awareness. You can then imagine that in the area beyond the field of consciousness, in the subconscious, there may be the remnants of past conflicts which, like magnets, try to prevent you from going inside to the centre. This may express itself as the 'one more time syndrome' (see p. 115); or whenever you want to go inside, images, memories or bad feelings from the subconscious grab your attention. You then have two options. The first is to try harder with your spiritual practice. Often you will find that those interferences then gradually disappear. The other option is that you have to do some psychotherapy work to 'de-energise' those subconscious blocks.

If you decide to go and see a psychotherapist, make sure that you continue with your spiritual practice as well. And, ideally, see a psychotherapist who has a spiritual perspective. Using Fig. 9 as an illustration, we can assume that a spiritually orientated psychotherapist would be using energies or elements from the superconscious in order to work on issues in the subconscious. That means that the subconscious issues get addressed and softened from two sides – from the field of conscious awareness and from the area of superconscious energies.

An example would be the 'bi-focal' vision of a psychosynthesis psychotherapist. In psychosynthesis therapists are trained to see both ego struggles and 'journey of the soul' issues in a client. The question of 'Which soul issue is trying to express itself through the presenting ego-problem?' would always be considered in therapy.

Being on a spiritual path is very precious and very important. See it as a gift that you don't want to lose.

Working with the Breath

Meditation and working with the breath help us to get ourselves unstuck and to make the connection with our higher Self . We withdraw life energy from the senses, which are attached to the multitude of sense objects that keep us trapped in the greenhouse. But rather than breaking through the walls that surround us, we withdraw inside to our centre (the 'I') and then draw the energy up the spine. The movement is in and up to a different dimension, to the level of the higher Self.

In yoga and Ayurveda this process is called 'pratyahara' (withdrawing energy from the senses) and 'pranayama'. Prana is the vital force, and pranayama means 'expansion of the vital force'. Pranayama is closely connected with slowing down and expanding the breath. This then slows down the mind and facilitates meditation. Paramahansa Yogananda teaches a pranayama technique called 'Kriya Yoga', which is a combination of pratyahara and pranayama:

FIG. 11: PRATYAHARA AND PRANAYAMA

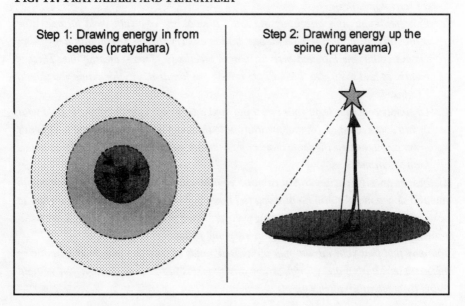

Step 1: Drawing energy in from senses (pratyahara)

Step 2: Drawing energy up the spine (pranayama)

The life force, which is ordinarily absorbed in maintaining heart action, must be freed for higher activities by a method of calming and stilling the ceaseless demands of the breath ... The *Kriya Yogi* mentally directs his life energy to revolve upward and downward, around the six spinal centers ... Through gradual and regular increase of the simple and foolproof methods of *Kriya*, man's body becomes astrally transformed day by day, and is finally fitted to express the infinite potentials of cosmic energy, which constitutes the first materially active expression of Spirit ... *Kriya* practice ... is accompanied from the very beginning by feelings of peace and by soothing sensations of regenerative effect in the spine. The ancient yogic technique converts the breath into mind-stuff. [76]

Try the following basic meditative breathing exercises.[77] They will most probably slow down your breath and induce a state of relaxation. But please note that breathing exercises and meditation, and especially Kriya Yoga are quite a sophisticated genre. It takes commitment, regular practice and a good teaching programme to fully benefit from it. In Chapter 11 you will find the MindBalancing meditation exercise, which you can use as a basic meditation programme. Further information and contact addresses are in 'Advice and Resources'.

BREATHING EXERCISES

For these exercises sit in the meditation posture as described in Chapter 3 under 'ideal sitting position'. Ideally you should do a relaxation and / or stretching exercise before sitting down in meditation posture.

1. *Concentrate on your breathing and count seven on the in-breath, hold for a count of three, a count of seven on the outbreath, hold for a count of three, and so on. Do this for several minutes.*
2. *Concentrate on your breathing and count nine on the in-breath, hold for one, nine counts on the out-breath, hold for one, and so on. Try this for several minutes.*
3. *Or just count one hundred breaths. One – breathe in. Two – breathe out. Three – breathe in and so on. Do this until you reach one hundred, by which time you should be relaxed.*
4. *Or simply concentrate on your breathing, and breathe in to the count of 10, hold your breath to the count of 10, and breathe out to the count of 10. You can use a higher or lower count, but use the same number for inhalation, holding and exhalation. Do this for a few minutes.*

All these breathing exercises aim at calming your breath, and when you calm your breath you also slow down the mind. Once you feel that your breathing has slowed down, try to just observe your breathing. By focusing your attention on your breathing you are withdrawing energy from the senses, and you are going inside.

You may find that your mind comes up with all kinds of thoughts to distract you during this exercise. That's quite normal. Allow any thoughts just to flow through you without giving them too much attention.

The Pendulum

Spirituality came to him rather late in life. But then, he seems to have taken his time with everything after the shock and subsequent struggle of his premature birth. Nevertheless, his life turned into a succession of great highs and great lows – university, extensive foreign travel, career, relationships with women, achievements and even glimpses of fame. Then gradually the lows were becoming more permanent, and the conviction that a new high was just around the corner weakened. The suspicion that he would never get out of a particular low increased in frequency and in strength. Alcohol, marijuana and sex became methods of trying to achieve yet another high or of trying to avoid or soften a low. He didn't know that drugs, drink and sex in excess are poison for the soul. They enslaved his will to the body, and they ultimately paralysed his will. All his attempts to get out of the lows or to maintain the highs were beginning to have the opposite effect of dragging him further down. Eventually he joined a new-age group and he began to have highs again. This time through guided imagery, emotional catharsis, and group sharings. By then his addictions had become quite well established as part of his life. For a few years he would spend his weekends on workshops and group-experiences, while during the week the drinking in the pub after work would continue. His relationships with women continued to be full of drama and destructiveness. Eventually full-blown depression set in. Anti-depressants further immobilised his will and even drove him slightly mad. After a suicide attempt he ended up in a psychiatric hospital. Finally he could hear his soul screaming. Finally he was ready for a spiritual path.

This is how it seems to be for many people. They need to hit 'rock bottom' first, before they can leave the legacies of the past behind and move on spiritually. Unfortunately some hit rock bottom and break their neck in the process. It does not have to be like this, but some people seem only to learn from the big crises, not from the smaller ones. This gives us the material for the pendulum model. Notice that the pendulum chart in Fig. 12 can be seen as a two-dimensional view of the three-dimensional egg, where S is the higher Self and M is the I.

In the world of duality we are sitting on the arm of a pendulum that swings between pleasure and pain, weakness and strength, happiness and sadness. The stronger the contrast between the opposites is (between A and B in Fig. 12), the stronger the swing of the pendulum will be, and the more we need to hold on to it while it swings (otherwise we would fall off). If the pendulum is stationary at A and we want to keep it there, we need use our strength to hold the arm to prevent it from swinging back towards M. When it is stationary at B we will want to give it a good push to swing it all the way back to A. All the while we are missing and avoiding M, which is the position of stillness for the pendulum.

We hardly have a chance to get up to the star (the higher Self) while the pendulum arm is swinging or stuck at either A or B. We obviously have most opportunity to climb up to the star when the pendulum is resting at M. Even a reduced swing from A1 to B1 could help us to start the climb.

Being stuck in pain (B) can also be connected with physical disease, possibly

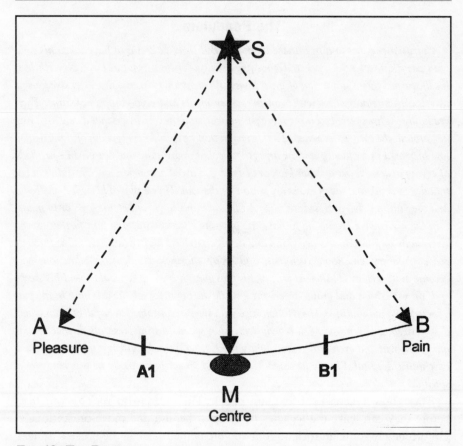

FIG. 12: THE PENDULUM

as a result of excessive and prolonged indulgence in sense pleasures (A). Then disease can be a spiritual opportunity. 'Disease may be a sign of wrong action in life, but it can also be an indication that the soul is directing energy within'.[78] Hence stuckness in B can indicate the soul's attempt to get to M (and from there to S).

Table 3 illustrates four different categories of paths. Many people come under category 3; they want to slow down. Their physical or mental health might force them to slow down. However, this slowing down will not stop the longing of the mind for habitual sense pleasures, habitual highs and lows. The highs and lows may just feel out of reach. Such a natural slowing down is usually meant to occur in mid-life. In a way it is an opportunity to withdraw energy from the senses and from the greenhouse set-up. But in our culture this is seen as mid-life crisis. It is not surprising that with increasing speed and intensifying sense stimulation many young people cannot keep up with the pace and present prematurely with midlife crisis 'symptoms'. I certainly experience this in my practice. Whole industries of personal fitness, travel, fashion etc. are cultivating their market of older people

	Journey	Process	Techniques	Pitfalls/ advantages
1	A - M and B - M	Centring and Withdrawing energy from the senses	Relaxation Disidentification	First stage of spiritual path Goal might still be unclear
	A1 - M and B1 - M	Going inside from a position, where the swinging of the pendulum is already reduced	Awareness Work on ego 'Greenhouse' work	Can be a necessary and positive move from enforced slowing down through illness or other life events
2	M - S	Spiritual path	Meditation, yoga, devotion	Requires work and discipline
3	A - A1 and B - B1	Slowing down	Relaxation techniques and cognitive therapy techniques	Can easily speed up again, especially when the need to slow down is resisted
4	A - S and B - S	Spiritual emergency; spirituality out of crisis - too much pleasure or too much pain	Grounding work and psychotherapy might be needed	Can be enforced spirituality; person not prepared for it and doesn't want it. But can be ok if work on ego is done subsequently
	A1 - S and B1 - S	Here at least from a slowed down position, but similar to A-S and B-S		

TABLE 3: THE SPIRITUAL JOURNEY

who desperately want to keep the pendulum swinging, even though their body, mind and soul say otherwise.

I have labelled category 4 *spiritual emergency*. This would refer to someone who has a sudden spiritual breakthrough or a spontaneous transpersonal experience without having the abilities, knowledge or ego-strength to understand and process the experience. One could speculate that this may apply to some patients in psychiatric hospital. In our pendulum model the direct moves from A, A1, B, B1 to S come under this category. This can be a rush towards the higher Self out of over-excitement of the senses or out of boredom (A – S); or it can be purely out of stuckness in pain and depression (B – S). This is always problematic and unlikely to be stable if the move to M, the stilling of the mind and the senses does not happen first of all. It is certainly better from A1 and B1, because some stilling will have already occurred.

Categories 1 and 2 describe the path that we have been following in this book, and which has been illustrated with the three-dimensional egg diagram.

YOUR PENDULUM (REFLECTION 10)

In this reflection I'd like you to apply the pendulum model to your life, in order to further clarify your pattern and to ascertain where you are now and what your next steps on the spiritual path could be.

Remember times of extreme pleasure, and times of extreme pain. How did you try to remain in the pleasure state and get out of the pain state? Did you ever try to climb up to the star from either of those states? Do you remember the swinging from A to B?

Remember times of stuck-ness in either A or B. Did you get bored with too much pleasure? How did you try to unstick yourself?

What pattern is operating in your life now? Do you need to reduce the swing of the pendulum? Do you need to unstick yourself?

Make plans for your path, and be very concrete about it. Be very detailed about your next steps – why, how, when, with whose help, teaching, advice.

11

Going In

This is the last chapter of the book. Most of the preceding ones have been full of models and maps to guide you away from the sense-mind towards the inner mind of the soul. In order to follow some of the maps you probably had to engage your intellect. I sincerely hope that some of it has given you a different understanding of yourself and the world you live in. But here is the catch: you cannot deeply change your thoughts through your thinking alone. For this you need meditation and the breath. The outer mind is just too powerful an instrument. It can easily hi-jack even good spiritual intentions and turn them into serving the ego. For example, you might be doing a regular meditation practice; then, after a while, the thought occurs: 'I am getting really good at this. I am much better than all those poor people who don't have a spiritual practice.' That would be an example of how the outer mind can try to turn your spiritual practice into something that benefits the ego. This is why devotion is such an important and necessary element in spiritual practice. Devotion is a wonderful safeguard against ego-inflation because it contains, or leads to, humility and compassion.

Devotion

Meditation and devotion belong together. This is a difficult point to argue, because devotion is another one of those touchy subjects. It sounds like submission, surrender, giving up our individuality, our free will. It sounds weak and whiney. But it is not. The opposite is true. Consider the attachments and addictions to the objects of the senses that have brought you problems and misery along the way, and will continue to do so. Those attachments are the devotion of the ego and the sense-mind. If you want to follow a spiritual path you need to be devoted to the soul, to God, and you can only do that when you let go of the attachments of the ego. The 'going inside' process that is advocated in this book means letting go of attachments and addictions to get to the soul-expression of those qualities – and that is devotion. Devotion is both, something that emerges in that process of letting go, and it can also help you with that process.

Here we also need to understand the difference between bhakti yoga (the yoga of devotion) and jnana yoga (the yoga of knowledge). Both are part of the Hindu religion and are two of the paths to enlightenment. In the teachings of Paramahansa Yogananda they are integrated, and Vivekananda too describes them as two of the four paths of yoga. This book, for example, is overtly jnana, because it addresses your intellect and tries to change your cognitions, the way you see things. But between the lines, this book also contains bhakti elements, because my intention in writing it comes from the heart and it tries to speak to your heart. Here is a definition:

Bhakti yoga is the practice of devotional disciplines, worship, prayer, chanting and singing with the aim of awakening love in the heart and opening oneself to God's grace.[79]

Why then might devotion be such a touchy subject for us Westerners? Mike King[80] suggests that the Western Christian tradition has emphasised bhakti at the expense of jnana, and that the Western focus on scientific knowledge might be a result of our repressed jnana-needs – a kind of backlash. It makes sense that from that emotional angle we feel uncomfortable with devotion. It feels like we have moved beyond something which deep down appears primitive. At the same time we have created a situation where the emotionality of the lower realms – like greed, anger, competitiveness – dominates so much of our lives.

But if we go back to the psychological greenhouse model, we can easily see that all those qualities of the higher unconscious like love, peace and beauty are somehow connected with devotion. So, could devotion be necessary for us to break away from our greenhouse space, to go beyond the materialism and emotionality that clogs up our psyche, to re-connect with our higher Self?

A second important point here is our attachment to emotions. As the higher qualities have been materialised or dragged down from the higher realms (see Fig. 5) or de-bhaktied, our soul-need for devotion has been looking for substitutes and has found them in the attachments to emotions and the false bliss that can be felt through sense gratification.

It is important to realise that there does not need to be a conflict between devotion and knowledge. What is needed is a balance of the two. This book tries to speak from this point of balance.

It is also very difficult to meditate just to clear the mind. It is much better to meditate from the heart. When you meditate from the heart you will feel devotion. Devotion to all the qualities of the superconscious, like love, compassion, peace, joy. Devotion is the energy that goes out from the heart to reach the qualities of the soul. It is like a beam. Devotion and compassion are also the soul qualities that help us transform the emotional turmoil of the ego.

Devotion is a quality of the soul. It is the soul's sense of one-ness with spirit. The soul is always and always has been in complete union with spirit. This is the no-boundary situation, the state beyond fragmentation and individuality, the state beyond alienation and separation.

This sense of unity and one-ness is present in us even in our incarnated ego state in the world of duality. The soul's craving often comes through as the ego's attachment to things and people. This could be seen as a twisted form of devotion. We become devoted to the fragments of the world of matter to the point of addiction. But our capacity to become devoted (addicted in the negative ego state) is essentially a soul quality. Similarly, many so-called neurotic states can be seen as very strong expressions of essential soul qualities. In OCD (obsessive compulsive disorder) it is the need for perfection, predictability, trust; in anxiety states the need for peace, calmness, no threats; and in depression it is the need for happiness and bliss.

Remember Richard's craving for perfection in Chapter 3? The main point in his therapy in the end was that he learnt to meditate. He learnt to detach himself from the strong emotions that his internal worrier were causing in him; and as a second step he began to acknowledge that it was his soul's craving for perfection that was really behind it all. Consequently he was able to direct his need for perfection to where it belonged – into meditation and spirituality. As a result he was able to function again as a manager without having to project his need for perfection into an imperfect world.

It is similar with devotion. Devotion is *the* essential soul quality, just as attachment and addiction are devotion's most troublesome manifestations in the world of the ego. Earlier on we explored the connection between attachments and the hungry baby syndrome. Hungry babies crave for love. Devotion and love are the same.

> Most psychological problems are based upon a lack of love in life. Love is the force that makes life worth living.[81]

But just as with perfection, fearlessness and happiness, ego gets it wrong with love as well. Love is said to the most important force in our universe. Love is a quality of the soul and a quality of God. When we love another person it is the God within us that loves the God within the other person. This love connection is often there at the beginning of relationships. But then it gradually gets perverted by the ego's needs for attachment, and Godly love becomes polluted with demands, jealousy, neediness, fear.

Yogananda says that we are all lost children, that we cannot find real love as long as we are disconnected from God's love. There is a sense of relief in this. The relief of not having to chase the 'perfect love' in human partners, or in romance, sex, or possessions any longer. But then this realisation can also create fear. Most of us have spent most of our lives trying to fill that gaping hole inside by searching for the ideal circumstances that would make life perfect. Our energy has gone into relationships, careers, mortgages, the accumulation of goods. We experience our striving as normal, because that's what everyone else seems to be doing. Life seems to be about finding the perfect love. Yogananda says 'you're looking in the wrong place'.

When we begin to detach from the world of matter through meditation, we begin to move towards soul and spirit. In this process the experience of one-ness gradually moves us from attachment and greed to a purer sense of love and devotion. By consciously using the soul quality of devotion in our meditation and in our daily lives, we support the process.

How then can we express devotion, especially if we feel rather uncomfortable with the idea? The divine can be worshipped in many different names or forms. Whether it is as father, mother, friend does not really matter. Most religions use a personalised form of God because it creates the most direct relationship. However, you might find the following suggestions easier:

> If the whole idea of a personal God is inconceivable to you, then throw out all form. Concentrate on Infinite Bliss, Infinite Intelligence, Omnipresent Consciousness, if such is more plausible to you. ...
> Think of God not as a word, or as a stranger, or as someone on high, waiting to judge and punish you. Think of Him as you would want to be thought of if you were God.[82]

I find this last suggestion particularly useful, because what we are really after is to connect with the divinity within ourselves. Once we are able to make this inner connection, then we can see divinity in and beyond all things. We can then even love ourselves in a soul-directed way.

Let us summarise:

1   Devotion is the highest soul quality that expresses transpersonal love to the God in ourselves and in all creation and beyond creation.
2   Devotion is the soul equivalent of the addictions and attachments of the ego in the greenhouse world.
3   Transformation of our addictions and attachments leads us to devotion to the divine.
4   We should consciously use devotion as a heart energy in and outside of meditation to connect with the divine, which is in and beyond matter.
5   Being on a spiritual path without devotion carries the pitfalls of ambition and pride. Devotion to a personal ideal of God evokes a natural inclination towards humility and service.

Devotion is not just a religious ritual, but can also be a very practical healing device. The 12-step programme, for example, was originally developed by Alcoholics Anonymous, and has been very successful in their world-wide movement. It is now also used by a wide range of groups dealing with sexual addictions, eating disorders, drug addictions, relationship problems, in short the wide range of sense addictions. These are the 12 steps, that are worked through in regular group meetings:

1   *We admitted we were powerless over addictive behaviour – that our lives had become unmanageable.*
2   *We came to believe that a power greater than ourselves could restore us to sanity.*
3   *We made a decision to turn our will and our lives over to the care of God as we understood God.*
4   *We made a searching and fearless moral inventory of ourselves.*
5   *We admitted to God, to ourselves, and to another human being the exact nature of our wrongs.*
6   *We were entirely ready to have God remove all these defects of character.*
7   *We humbly asked God to remove our shortcomings.*
8   *We made a list of all persons we had harmed and became willing to make amends to them all.*
9   *We made direct amends to such people wherever possible, except when to do so would injure them or others.*
10   *We continued to take personal inventory and when we were wrong promptly admitted it.*
11   *We sought through prayer and meditation to improve our conscious contact with God as we understood God, praying only for knowledge of God's will for us and the power to carry that out.*
12   *Having had a spiritual awakening as the result of these steps, we tried to carry this message to other addicts and to practise these principles in our lives.*

These twelve steps cover the areas of self-analysis, letting go of sense attachments, connecting with soul, letting go of the past, and even devotion. We can use the steps, or at least some of them, as guidelines for our journey away from sense attachments towards soul.

Having now followed the maps in this book through the jungle of the world of maya you are now coming to the 'doing part' – the practice of going inside. The maps have hopefully shown you that the only way out is in; now you are beginning to go in.

When you begin to work on yourself, you need to be very clear about why you would want to do that. Stilling the mind and withdrawing energy from the senses are the very central things you need to do. This is a process of self-healing that you will be starting. The *why* is important, because on the path of withdrawing energy from the sense-mind and the ego, they will fight back. They will try to regain their lost territory. I gave a few examples in the section on the one more time syndrome. There are many more. The greenhouse world is full of rational justifications why this going inside business is completely un-natural, even perverse. The following contrary statements are quite likely to come up in your mind or from other people:

It is human nature to be greedy, envious, competitive etc.
It is in our genes to be like this or that.
We have inherited this or that from our animal past.
We have inherited this or that from our parents.
Look at him or her; they have found happiness through this or that.
Look at this or that famous person; they have made it without meditating.

All those statements come from the ego trying to hold on to its territory. The earlier chapters should have given you some ammunition to fight back. However, you might need a spiritual counsellor or like-minded friends to discuss some of those counter-attacks from the ego. But first and foremost you need to be clear why you want to spiritualise your life. Obviously, if you have started on a spiritual path out of a deep crisis, i.e. your pendulum was stuck in either pain or pleasure, you will initially know exactly why you want to change your life. But do not be fooled. As soon as you are beginning to feel better, the old habits will try to re-claim their space.

YOUR SPIRITUAL PATH (REFLECTION 11)

Try to answer the question why you would want to be on a spiritual path.

Look back over your life pattern, and try to discover in it, like a thread, your soul's journey back to spirit. Just assume for a moment that this life of yours was set as a lesson in a classroom. What has been the theme of your lesson throughout your life? What would that theme say about the hurdles that you have needed to overcome in order to connect with soul and spirit? Can you now, at this point in your life, affirm to yourself that you have struggled enough with the lesson, and that you now need to move on?

Also become aware of how your ego might fight back. What emotional and behavioural habits have always persisted or come back in the past? What excuses or justifications would you expect your mind to come up with?

Meditation

This chapter introduces a programme of relaxation and meditation that I call MindBalancing. This practical programme brings together all the different strands from the previous chapters. Steps One, Two and Three of the programme are also available on audio-cassette (see 'Advice and Resources' for details). The exercises in steps One and Two have grown out of my work with individuals and groups, and they are based on some of my previously published work.[83] But here they are developed further to serve the purpose of the book, and they are preparation exercises for meditation. The meditation (Step Three in the programme) is an introduction to meditation as concentration. It is a technique that you can use to go beyond the fragmentation and busy-ness of the outer mind to that place of stillness within, from manas to buddhi. There are many other meditation techniques and programmes – there is a whole world out (or in) there. Meditation is a sacred practice to connect with the divine. Many of the techniques are ancient and very powerful, and they require disciplined practice under guidance. The meditation exercise suggested here is a good starting point, and it is tried and safe. If you want to go further, you will find some suggestions in the 'Advice and Resources' section at the end.

MindBalancing Practice

In the ultimate sense, all things are made of pure consciousness; their finite appearance is the result of the relativity of consciousness. Therefore, if you want to change anything in yourself, you must change the process of thought that occasions the materialization of consciousness into different forms of matter and action. That is the way, the only way, to remold your life.[84]

INTRODUCTION

The theme throughout this book has been how you can change your mind. The previous chapters have given you models and maps for the journey from the sense-mind to the intelligence of the soul, from intellect to intelligence, from outer mind to inner mind, or from manas to buddhi. With the models and maps so far, we have mainly spoken to your outer mind in order to re-assure your intellect that it is all right to redress the balance in favour of the inner mind. We first of all need the outer mind's co-operation, before we can slow it down, still it, in order to then gradually operate more from the inner mind which is our true centre. So far this book has been about preparing the way to re-dress the balance by introducing to you a new philosophy, a new understanding of who you are and who you might be. We have now reached a point on the path, where I should like to introduce the MindBalancing practice, which consists of a series of reflections and relaxation and meditation exercises. These exercises will help more directly to shift your inner balance towards the intelligence of your soul (your wisdom or intuition). David Frawley emphasises how important such a shift is for all of us:

Our modern information-sensation culture is dominated by the outer mind and lacking in intelligence. We are more concerned with gathering information through the mind than with digesting it, which requires intelligence. We have developed many ways to expand the field of sensory data, but not the wisdom to use it properly.[85]

It may be helpful if, at this stage, you re-connect with what you have learnt from working through the book so far. The purpose throughout has been to make some doors visible in your outwardly orientated sense-mind, to create some flexibility in the way you view your life and your world, to draw maps for the journey to the inner mind, which is the intelligence of the soul. Perhaps you could re-visit those doors and those markers on your map by looking back at the reflections in the previous chapters. Or you may want to just look back at what you may have underlined or written down while you have been reading. You are on a journey, and anything that can illuminate your path will help.

STRUCTURED ANALYSIS

Throughout this book we have been pleading with your outer mind or intellect to allow this process of going within to happen. At this point I should like to suggest a practice that may satisfy your intellect, and may help you to develop a different, but still very rational, attitude towards the thoughts and emotions of the outer mind. The practice originates in a school of therapy called cognitive-behavioural therapy. Although this therapy is often dismissed as being superficial and non-spiritual, I have found that many of the techniques are quite similar to what would be used in yogic and Ayurvedic counselling. David Frawley in a chapter on 'Ayurvedic Counseling and Behavioral Modification' says:

> Ayurvedic counseling is very practical and involves various prescriptions for changing how we live. Meeting with an Ayurvedic counselor involves reviewing the results of implementing these prescriptions, and is done in a consistent step-by-step manner. Ayurvedic counseling is educational in nature. The therapist helps the client learn how the mind and body work so that we can use them properly. The patient is a student. Therapy is a learning process. Ayurveda looks upon someone suffering from a psychological problem not as a bad or disturbed person, but as someone who does not understand how to use the mind properly.[86]

An extended version of the following exercise, which I call a structured analysis is also available on audio cassette as part of my cassette pack *Anxiety and Stress Management Toolkit*[87] (see 'Advice and Resources' for details). You may find that this exercise becomes easier once you can do it in connection with a relaxation technique. You can use one of the breathing exercises from p. 132 for this, or Steps One and Two of the MindBalancing practice further on.

• Part One: The Triggers

Remember a recent occasion when you felt anxious, depressed, stressed, upset. Or you may want to use one of the 'greenhouse qualities', that particularly bothers you, from p. 100. Identify as far as possible the day, time, and location of the start of the feeling(s) by scanning back through time. Do this by closing your eyes and going back in time bit by bit.

Once you have identified the situation when and where the feeling started, vividly imagine yourself in that situation just before the feeling started. Picture yourself, the surroundings, other people, the sounds and smells, the temperature.

Then try and be yourself in that situation. What was it like to be in that particular situation? What did you experience?

What were you doing or saying?

What were others doing or saying?

What were your feelings?

What physical sensations did you experience?

What thoughts were going through your mind?

Did you remember something from the past?

Did you anticipate something in the future?

You may find it a bit unpleasant to remember everything in so much detail. Or you may find that there are blocks to remembering. Your mind may drift into thinking about other things. Keep your body and especially your breathing calm and relaxed, and gently guide your mind back to the situation.

Once you have explored the context of the beginning of the feelings, see if you can get a sense of what may have been the trigger(s). This may not be very clear-cut, and perhaps it seems as if there was no trigger, as if it all happened 'out of the blue'. If that's the case, focus especially on the things that you did not want to remember, or the things that you had forgotten and only just remembered. Also look at the situation as a whole: Was the constellation similar to ones that you have found difficult in the past? Is there a pattern that goes back a long way?

Now make some notes about what you have found out about the trigger(s) of those feelings.

• Part Two: The Event
Now go back to remembering the situation. But this time focus on your experience of the anxiety, depression or other feeling or quality that you have chosen.

Then try and be yourself in that situation. What was it like to be in that particular situation? What did you experience?

See if you can get a sense of what your feelings were trying to tell you. Was it a message from the past? How relevant is that message now?

Again, make some notes about your exploration.

• Part Three: The Conclusion
Now go to the point in time when the anxiety, depression, or other feeling stopped or changed (if it did). What were the circumstances under which it changed? Did it have anything to do with anything you did, said, thought or felt? Did it have anything to do with other people's actions?

Make notes.

Look at the three sets of notes you have made during this exercise and apply the following criteria to them:

1. What can you learn from the information? How could you summarise the information?

2. What is your 'gut reaction' to the notes and the reflection in general?

3. Is there an image or symbol for you as a result of this exercise? Draw it if you want to.

This practice will help you to learn that unpleasant thoughts and feelings usually do not come out of the blue. Often we just do not remember the triggers, because they are part of old and well-established unconscious patterns, or the situation was so unpleasant that our memory was impaired by the level of distress. The results of your structured analysis may also give you some ideas as to where you might be able to interrupt the cycles of action and reaction by behaving differently, thinking differently, or by becoming more careful about the external influences to which you expose yourself. The steps of the MindBalancing Meditation further on will teach you techniques that you can employ to interrupt those cycles.

DEVELOPING SATTVA

> Good is the steadfastness whereby a man
> Masters his beats of heart, his very breath
> Of life, the action of his senses; fixed
> In never-shaken faith and piety:
> That is of *Sattwan*, Prince! 'soothfast' and fair!
> Stained is the steadfastness whereby a man
> Holds to his duty, purpose, effort, end,
> For life's sake, and the love of goods to gain,
> Arjuna! 'tis of *Rajas*, passion-stamped!
> Sad is the steadfastness wherewith the fool
> Cleaves to his sloth, his sorrow, and his fears,
> His folly and despair. This – Pritha's son! -
> Is born of *Tamas*, 'dark' and miserable![88]

Sattva has been mentioned in Chapter 2 as an important element in yogic and Ayurvedic cosmology. It is the universal quality of stability, harmony and virtue. The other two gunas are rajas, which is turbulence, passion and activity, and tamas, which is heaviness, darkness and dullness. The gunas as primal qualities are the energetic origin of the grosser forms of creation like the elements.

The mind is also composed of the three gunas. The aim of psycho-spiritual development is to increase sattva in the mind as a return to peace and harmony. This is not as simple as it may sound and it depends very much on our starting point, i.e. which guna is predominant in us to start with. If tamas is the predominant mental energy, then rajas will probably initially have to be increased before sattva can become the goal. An example would be someone who is depressed, lethargic and self-destructive, in other words, very tamasic. Someone like that would first of all need to become wilful and possibly develop some of the rajasic qualities of ambition, anger and agitation before the sattvic qualities of enlightenment, compassion and enthusiasm can be on the agenda.

The three gunas of sattva, rajas and tamas are the most important qualities that define our mental state.

> To have Sattva predominant in our nature is the key to health, creativity and spirituality. Sattvic people possess an harmonious and adaptable nature which gives the greatest freedom from disease, both physical and mental. ... Rajasic people have good energy but burn themselves out through excessive activity. Their minds are usually agitated and seldom at peace. ... Tamasic types have deep-seated psychological blockages. Their energy and emotion tend to be stagnant and repressed, and they do not know what their problems really are.[89]

It is vital for us to shift our mental energy towards sattva if we want to balance mind and body. From the definition of the gunas and from the discussion of our world of splitting and fragmentation, it becomes obvious that we live in very rajasic times. In a way we can apply the pendulum model (see p. 134) by understanding how we often swing from rajas to tamas and back again – times of hyperactivity are often followed by times of lethargy and stagnation.

Meditation is obviously connected with sattva. But a sattvic state cannot be achieved with meditation alone. Other lifestyle and attitude changes are also necessary. The Mental Constitution Chart on p.149 will give you some idea about your mental constitution, and also point out areas for you that might need some work.

> Generally one Guna predominates in our nature. However, we all have spiritual or sattvic moments, rajasic or disturbed periods, and tamasic or dull times which may be shorter or longer depending upon our nature. We also have sattvic. rajasic or tamasic phases of life which may last for months or even years.[90]

In the chart the left column is sattva, the middle one rajas, and the right one tamas. Tick what applies to you for each item and then total the ticks for each column. Most of us, in our present culture, probably have a predominance of rajas. According to Frawley the chart also gives some indication about our susceptibility for psychological problems, where more tamas means more psychological issues, and more sattva means a balanced mind.

Many of the items in the chart can be understood with the models and maps that have been introduced throughout this book. Perhaps you could go through the items and check your understanding why each one might be sattvic or tamasic.

MINDBALANCING MEDITATION

Meditation techniques all, in a way, aim at the meditator detaching from the sense-mind to get to the inner mind. The details of meditation practice depend on the school of meditation that you follow. There is the contemplative prayer of the Christian Carmelite tradition, and there are many different Buddhist and Hindu ways. You need to find the way that feels right for you, or that speaks to you. Once you have found your way, however, it is important that you stick to it and follow it with determination and discipline and devotion. Endless searching, and changing from one way to another, can be yet another skilful strategy of the ego trying to avoid the journey to the soul.

Ultimately meditation is best without form, without images, so that the space becomes open for spirit, open for the soul's connection with God. It is therefore important not to confuse the guided imagery techniques, which are widely used in different psycho-spiritual schools and in new-age movements, with true meditation. However, it is usually not advisable to try and just empty the mind, because this 'may be no more than to put our attention into our subconscious, where its dark tendencies can further inflict their pain upon us'.[92] Another way of looking at this is shown in Figures 9 and 11 (see p. 127 and p. 131). They show that when we go within to that centre in a two-dimensional way, we are still surrounded by the subconscious and its energies. We need to do it three-dimensionally – the in *and* up movement, illustrated in Step 2 of Fig. 11 – in order to detach from the influence of the subconscious. It means that we are connecting our inner Self with a higher power that can hold us and protect us from the dark energies of the subconscious.

In this context devotion, as discussed earlier, becomes an important protective element for meditation practice. David Frawley, for example, suggests the use of mantra (sacred words or sounds) to prepare the ground for meditation. He even goes as far as saying:

> It can be far more helpful to regularly chant a mantra than to analyze our psychological problems. The mantra changes the energetic structure of the mind which dissolves the problem, while thinking about the problem can reinforce it.[93]

Sound and breath go together, and both are closely connected with the mind. The breathing exercises may have given you some understanding of how slowing the breath can also slow down the mind. We are now going further by combining many of the elements from this book into a self-development routine that you can use as a regular practice for relaxation, energisation, concentration and meditation. The concentration-meditation part of the routine also contains pranayama and mantra, so that you can use it as a preparation for formless meditation, which

MENTAL CONSTITUTION CHART[91]

Diet	Vegetarian	Some Meat	Heavy Meat Diet
Drugs, Alcohol, Stimulants	Never	Occasionally	Frequently
Sensory Impressions	Calm, Pure	Mixed	Disturbed
Need for Sleep	Little	Moderate	High
Sexual Activity	Low	Moderate	High
Control of Senses	Good	Moderate	Weak
Speech	Calm & Peaceful	Agitated	Dull
Cleanliness	High	Moderate	Low
Work	Selfless	For Personal Goals	Lazy
Anger	Rarely	Sometimes	Frequently
Fear	Rarely	Sometimes	Frequently
Desire	Little	Some	Much
Pride	Modest	Some Ego	Vain
Depression	Never	Sometimes	Frequently
Love	Universal	Personal	Lacking in Love
Violent Behavior	Never	Sometimes	Frequently
Attachment to Money	Little	Some	A lot
Contentment	Usually	Partly	Never
Forgiveness	Forgives easily	With Effort	Holds long term grudges
Concentration	Good	Moderate	Poor
Memory	Good	Moderate	Poor
Will Power	Strong	Variable	Weak
Truthfulness	Always	Most of the Time	Rarely
Honesty	Always	Most of the Time	Rarely
Peace of Mind	Generally	Partly	Rarely
Creativity	High	Moderate	Low
Spiritual Study	Daily	Occasionally	Never
Mantra, Prayer	Daily	Occasionally	Never
Meditation	Daily	Occasionally	Never
Service	Much	Some	None

Total   Sattva_____   Rajas_____   Tamas_____ should be practised under the guidance of a meditation teacher (see 'Advice and Resources' for a list of organisations). If you feel you want to use MindBalancing as a regular routine, you may find it easier to practice the relaxation, energisation and meditation using the MindBalancing tape (see 'Advice and Resources' for ordering information).

STEP ONE: MUSCULAR RELAXATION AND ENERGISATION

The following quote from Paramahansa Yogananda expresses how important muscular relaxation is for spiritual development. Exercise and hatha yoga postures will all help to relax the muscles. The muscular relaxation exercise in this part is a simple but effective way of first of all learning to recognise the difference between tension and relaxation in the different muscle groups, and then consciously to let go of tension and allow relaxation.

> Remember that muscular relaxation, though it is not easy, is extremely important for spiritual development. Muscular relaxation means withdrawing energy and consciousness from the wave of muscular motions.

Yogananda also says:

> The first knot to untie, in order to release the Spirit within, is the knot of muscular consciousness. It is necessary to remove all tension and send relaxation to the knots – big and small – in the muscles.[94]

In addition to relaxing your muscles, this exercise also has the effect of recharging your body with life energy. You may want to think of it as many tiny life energy channels that run through your body, and by relaxing your muscles you can open those channels so that life energy can flow more freely again.

Make sure you are sitting or lying down comfortably with your eyes closed. Have your arms by your side, and your legs uncrossed. Let your whole body relax. It is important that you do not worry how well you are doing with these exercises, because you will improve with regular practice.

Then, for each of the muscle groups that are listed below, take a deep breath in and tense the muscles in the way suggested, hold your breath and the muscular tension and concentrate on the tension. Hold breath and tension for five to ten seconds. And then let go of the breath and of the tension. While letting go, concentrate on the difference between tension and relaxation. Keep your breathing slow and shallow and let go of more tension from those muscles with your breath for another five to ten seconds, before you move on to the next muscle group. After the tense-relax sequence you may feel warmth or tingling in the muscles. Enjoy that as a sign of tension moving out.

- *Concentrate on your left hand, then right hand, by making a fist.*

- *Concentrate on your left arm, then right arm: clench your fist, bend your arm at the elbow, bringing your wrist up to your shoulder, and tense the upper and lower arm muscles (try to differentiate between upper and lower arm).*

- *This time stretch out first your left, then your right arm, clench the fist and tense upper and lower arm.*

- *Then shrug your shoulders, bringing them up to your ears, and concentrate on the tension in your shoulders and neck.*

- *Tense your neck by bending your head backward, concentrating on the tension in the front and back of your neck.*

- *Then bend your head forward.*

- *Concentrate on your face and tense the muscles in your face by squeezing your eyes shut, biting your teeth together and pressing your lips together.*

- *Concentrate on your lower abdomen and then upper abdomen by pulling those areas in (the upper abdomen and stomach area can be pulled in and up).*

- *Concentrate on your back by arching it.*

- *Concentrate on your buttocks by squeezing them together.*

- *Concentrate on your left leg, then right leg, and try to differentiate between foot, calf, and thigh. First lift your left leg with your toes pointing away from you, then with your toes pointing towards you. Then do the same with your right leg.*

- *Then take a deep breath in and hold it and tense your whole body at the same time. And then let go. Do this three times.*

- *And finally, take in a deep breath without holding it and throw the breath out again. The just wait for the in-breath to happen again. Enjoy the state of breathlessness before the in-breath happens. For a few moments just watch your breathing happening.*

STEP TWO: BREATHING RELAXATION

You can let this step follow on from Step One, or you can do each one of the two parts separately. On the tape they follow one-another. While your body is calm and relaxed, you can then relax the muscles of your body more by using your breathing. You can use this practice as regular relaxation. You will gradually acquire the skill to use your breath for calming yourself down whenever you feel tense. The breath, as we have repeatedly discussed throughout, is essential in meditation practice. With our breath we exchange energy with our environment – carbon dioxide goes out and oxygen comes in. In a way we take our environment in through our breath, and we go out into our environment with our breath. It is a constant rhythmic flow. This flow usually happens without our awareness, but we can become aware of it and then our breathing can become our ally in the meditative process of healing. The breath is also intimately connected with the life force (prana) and with the mind, especially with the emotions. Prana is said to be highly concentrated in oxygen, and the 'explosion' of oxygen atoms in the body releases prana and re-charges the body. When we slow down the breath, we also slow down the heart, the mind, and we slow down the process of decay in the body. There are also some specific breathing techniques (pranayama) that directly influence the flow of prana in the body.

Initially, do this exercise lying down (see p. 30 for the ideal lying position). But later on also try it sitting in your meditation posture. Have your eyes closed. Focus your full attention on your breathing and put your right hand on your stomach just above your waistline; monitoring your breathing with your right hand

Now take a few deep breaths and make sure your stomach comes out when you breathe in and that it goes in when you breathe out. Continue breathing regularly and calmly. Push your stomach out a little when you breathe in, and pull your stomach in a little bit when you breathe out. Your diaphragm expands when you breathe in to fill your lungs, and it contracts when you exhale..

Breathe in continuously and smoothly and then breathe out continuously and smoothly, without holding your breath. Keep your breathing regular and shallow, in and out through your nose.

Use the word RELAX as a mantra. Say RE to yourself when you breathe in and LAX when you breathe out. Make sure that you do not move your tongue or your mouth when you say RE – LAX to yourself. You can now remove your right hand from your stomach area, but put it back there when you feel you do not breathe with your diaphragm.

You are now focusing all your attention on your breathing and on the word RELAX. Through this concentration you are relaxing both body and mind.

You can now concentrate on different parts of your body, breathing into them and letting tension flow out from them with each breath out. If you find it difficult to imagine that you are breathing into different parts of your body, put your hand on your knee for a moment and let your breath flow into your knee. With your hand you may even notice a slight movement in your knee in rhythm with your breathing.

For 15-20 seconds each concentrate on the following body parts, breathing energy into those parts saying RE, and letting tension flow out from those parts on the out-breath saying LAX. Imagine that there is a tube that connects your breathing with those parts of your body, and the breath flows through that tube directly there and out from it:

- *Concentrate on your left hand, then right hand.*

- *Concentrate on your left arm, then right arm, and try to differentiate between upper and lower arm.*

- *Concentrate on your neck, front and back.*

- *Concentrate on your face.*

- *Concentrate on your lower abdomen and then upper abdomen.*

- *Concentrate on your back.*

- *Concentrate on your buttocks.*

- *Concentrate on your left leg, then right leg, and try to differentiate between foot, calf, and thigh.*

Now choose one particular part of your body for more relaxation. It may even be an organ or an area inside your body. Perhaps choose a part of your body that you are concerned about at the moment, or where you feels tension, pain or discomfort. Breathe into that part of your body and out from it saying RE-LAX in rhythm with your breathing.

You can finish this exercise with a few pranic breaths, which are breathing techniques that have an effect on particular forms of prana in body and mind. Many of my clients have found the following ones particularly useful. They are apana, which is the descending breath and helps in grounding, samana, which is the centring breath and good for balancing, and prana, which is energising and vitalising.[95]

- *Apana: Take a deep breath down to the bottom of your spine and hold it there. And then upon exhalation ground the energy downward through your feet into the earth. Release all physical and mental toxins into the ground. Do this five times.*

- *Samana: Now breathe down into the navel and imagine energy from the entire universe entering your body. Hold the breath firmly in the navel and let your digestive fire blaze up. On exhalation let the breath extend outward from the navel providing nourishment to all the tissues of your body and to your mind and heart. Do this five times.*

- *Prana: Now take a few deep breaths drawing the energy from the space around you to the point between the eyebrows. Hold the energy there upon retention and breathe out from that point. Imagine the energy coming in through all your senses and going out through all your senses, opening and purifying all the channels of your brain and mind.*

Perhaps you could use Yogananda's suggestion as a 'homework' to help you gradually carry an awareness of your breathing into your daily life:

Observe how breathing is affected by your surroundings, your thoughts, your actions. Conversely, scrutinise the thoughts and feelings generated in you by changes in the depth and rhythm of your breath.[96]

In order move on to Step Three of MindBalancing, you should have practised Steps One and Two regularly for a few weeks. In our MindBalancing groups we ask participants to practice Steps One and Two daily for two weeks, and do a structured analysis of emotional issues when needed, before moving on to Step Three. They also work through reading material from this book during that time. In weekly group meetings we share our experiences with the practices and the reading.

You need to develop some awareness of tension and relaxation in your body in everyday life, and you should learn to calm yourself down by just using your breath. First, try it out in non-demanding situations, like when driving the car, or when you are sitting and not doing much else. Some elements of Steps One and Two are easy to practise even in public places, like for example tensing up your whole body, briefly holding your breath and throwing it out, or breathing into different body parts, and silently saying RE-LAX to yourself in rhythm with your breathing. Then, gradually try consciously relaxing yourself in more demanding situations. But do not expect immediate success. The old habits and ways of reacting to pressure are usually quite strong, because they have developed over a long period of time.

STEP THREE: MINDBALANCING MEDITATION

He who conquers the mind, conquers the world.[97]

Meditation happens with the head and the heart. In yogic science the heart is the seat of consciousness. In terms of the chakras (energy centres along the spine) the heart centre is the centre for transpersonal love. The *third eye* is the point between the eyebrows, where you gaze with your eyes in meditation. It is the Christ-centre or the centre of will, from where life energy gets dispersed into the body. In meditation the third eye can be seen as the transmitter and the heart as the receiver of spiritual energies. Meditation opens the heart and focuses concentration and will from the third eye.

In this step you are using the skills you have learned in the previous steps, and you are learning meditation in order to withdraw energy from the outer mind and the senses so that you can be more in touch with your inner mind, your soul-mind. This meditation is a journey of you changing your mind. It is about going from your outer mind to your inner mind, to your true Self; your breath now becomes your guide on the journey.

Normally you are far away from your true Self. Activities, thoughts and feelings take all your attention. But behind, underneath and within all your actions, thoughts and feelings there is your true Self, which is calm, solid, and strong. It is like the vast stillness of the ocean beneath the ripples and the waves. That *you* is timeless and spaceless, but it is also with you, in every part of you at all times. You carry it around with you wherever you go, whatever you do.

In order to get to that inner you, you need to go beyond your thoughts and your feelings. You need to go to a much deeper part of your mind, beyond the mind that is constantly pre-occupied with thoughts, feelings and fantasies about external issues and events that usually belong to the past or the future.

Ponder for a moment that your whole reality is determined by the perceptions and the thinking of your outer mind. And your outer mind is structured by long-learnt patterns and subconscious tendencies. Hence the reality you are experiencing is made up by your very own outer mind and is therefore uniquely different from anyone else's reality.

I am suggesting that you can change your mind, because there is a you that is beyond your usual mind. There is a you that is beyond all the different layers of your thinking and your feeling. That you is the seer, the witness, your Self.

From that inner you, you can control your thinking, and by controlling your thinking you can also control your reality, even create a different reality.

You can see this process as a journey. The journey is from your usual experience of reality as being caught up with your work, your family and friends – all the things you do. You will make the first step on the journey by just sitting with your eyes closed. You are not doing anything apart from sitting with your eyes closed in silence.

What usually happens then is that your mind becomes busy inside – desperately trying to find things to do to replace the external stimuli that are shut off. Your mind may concentrate on sounds or on bodily sensations. It may be having thoughts about anything. In this meditation you are going to try to be a detached observer of all those thoughts and feelings that go through your mind.

The tools you have to avoid getting pulled into all this busy-ness of your mind are your attention and your breathing. Both your attention and your breathing are very close to that inner you, and they can guide you beyond all those thoughts, emotions and bodily sensations that rush through your mind.

Start off this meditation by focusing your attention on your breathing.

Watch how the breath enters your body through your nostrils, feeling cool when it touches the inside of your nostrils, and warm when it flows out – cool on the in-breath and warm on the out-breath.

Just watch the rhythm of your breathing and allow your breath to slow down. Let your attention follow the whole length of the wave of your breath.

While your attention is on the rhythm of your breathing, your breath slows down and the thoughts and the feelings of the outer mind also slow down. Your breath is the anchor for your concentration.

At regular intervals during this meditation put your full attention on your breathing, following the flow of your breath – in and out. Cool air coming in, warm air going out. While your attention is with your breath, also let your eyes behind your closed eyelids gaze upward to that point between the eyebrows without straining your eyes.

Whenever you notice that your attention has gone elsewhere, either to a sound, or a physical sensation, or a thought, bring it back to your breathing and make sure your eyes are gazing up to the point between your eyebrows. Try to be a detached observer of your thoughts, feelings and sensations.

Your breathing can serve as an anchor for your attention, because the mind and the breathing are closely connected. Concentrating on your breath internalises your mind. It also helps you to be in the present moment, breath by breath, moment by moment.

At times you may find that there is a particularly powerful thought, or a feeling like fear, or a physical sensation like tension that is trying to grab your attention. You can then do several things before you bring your attention back to your breathing:

1 *You can try to breathe into that thought or sensation. Breathing into it and breathing out from it – softening it. Do this several times and then bring your attention back to your breath and the point between the eyebrows.*

2 *Or you can concentrate on the coolness that remains in your nostrils during that brief pause at the end of the in-breath, just before the out-breath starts, and on the warmth at the end of the out-breath. In those brief moments of breathlessness, send the coolness from your nostrils to the thought or sensation, and let the warmth disperse out from it.*

3 *Or you can put the thought or feeling into space. Imagine putting the thought into the vast space that surrounds you, and that is also inside you. See the thought flowing in space. See it flowing away, dissolving in the vast inner and outer space that is our home.*

Then, with your attention settled in your breathing, use the mantra So-Hom in rhythm with your breathing. Say SO as you breathe in and HOM as you breathe out. So-Hom. Don't move your mouth or your tongue while you say So-Hom to yourself. Let your breath make the sound. Continue this meditation just with the mantra for a little while.

It is difficult to say how much time you should spend with each one of these three steps. On the tape Steps One and Two together are 30 minutes and Step Three is 30 minutes. If you are not using the tape, and you just memorise the instructions, then you should give yourself at least 20 minutes for Steps One and Two, and at least 15 minutes for Step Three. It is obviously easier to use the tape, because you then have an external time-keeper.

Your outer mind will, no doubt, ask what results you can expect from this practice. However, your inner mind will probably soon 'breathe a sigh of relief' for the regular moments of peace and stillness. It is not possible to say exactly what you will gain from meditation practice, because your starting point, your reality is unique. I can only speak from my experience and the experience of many other people that I know about, to give you some ideas about what may happen to you. Your life energy may become more centred, and as a result you will probably become calmer, your concentration will improve, and you will find a new and more blissful inner balance. You will most certainly be able to use the techniques of relaxation and breathing in everyday life to distance yourself from disturbing external influences, emotions and sensations. Be prepared that you may also become more sensitive and more compassionate, because at the level of the inner mind there is unity with everything and all.

You also need to be aware that old habits and patterns may want to sneak back in – the sense-mind fighting back. Throughout this book we have discussed some of the ways in which this might happen. Or life crises may throw you off your course again and again. Then you need to realise that life without conflict and crises is just not possible in our world of duality. However, there is a lot you can do. First of all, you can deal with crises as best as you can. Secondly, it is up to you how deeply you let any crisis or conflict affect you. And thirdly, you can see each crisis as a lesson that has come your way to teach you something. But most of all, you need to firmly know that there is a deeper reality within you and all around you – a reality that is beyond the ripples and waves of the outer mind.

Meditation may often feel like a battle for you. Whatever you do, the outer mind just will not calm down. The techniques may give you brief moments of peace, but before you can help it your whole being is propelled back into yet another one of your mind's infinite themes. Your resolve to withdraw your attention wanes. In addition your body might begin to ache. When that happens, do not stop right away. Keep struggling a bit further, a bit longer. The struggle is normal. It is like going to the gym – with the struggle you are exercising your inner mind and you are making it stronger. But don't get too tense about the struggle either. Always re-focus your mind on relaxation.

You may begin to feel like I sometimes do, when I drive along in my car and listen to the news on the radio. I see the busy-ness around me, and I hear more busy bits coming into my mind about all the exciting and disturbing things that are happening on our planet. Then there is this little strong voice in me that quite firmly says: 'All that is not real', and sometimes I can really feel that it is not real. Then I can sense that there is only a thin veil of outer reality, and behind that veil, just behind my vision, my hearing and my thinking there is a much bigger, much more real reality. I appreciate those moments when I can see or sense beyond the world of matter. That, I think, is what it may feel like for you when you are connected with your inner mind. When you are disconnected from that central you, and you are completely lost in the frantic movement of the outer mind, then the external busy-ness feels much more piercing, spinning the wheel of the mind ever faster.

There is now a growing body of research evidence showing that relaxation and meditation methods have a beneficial and healing effect on a wide range of psychological and physical disorders. You can, with confidence, affirm to yourself that the regular practice of the MindBalancing programme suggested on these pages will have a positive effect on your physical and mental health. Seen from a yogic perspective, meditation is the deepest form of healing. Nothing else can be healed without healing the mind first, because the mind, as the most subtle form of matter, is where the grosser forms of matter originate. By healing the mind we are healing its multitude of expression, e.g. the physical body, our relationships, our society and our planet. However, there are times when more direct physical forms of healing become necessary. There is a vast system of physical Ayurvedic healing, which has not been the theme of this book. It consists of diagnostic, dietary, lifestyle, herbal and other treatment methods, which are based in the same philosophy that this book is based in. The interested reader is referred to the 'Advice and Resources' below for further information.

The ultimate aim of meditation is to be in touch with that bigger reality, with God deep within you, and to operate in the outer world from that connected-ness. I hope that this book and the MindBalancing practice can be tools on your path. If you want to go further on the path and develop a regular spiritual discipline, then you need to find spiritual teachings that give you the methods and the inspiration that can guide you further. In 'Advice and Resources' you will find my recommendations as to where you could look for that.

If you use intuition, you will know the very purpose for which you exist in this world; and when you find that, you find happiness. ... The only way to know and to live in truth is to develop the power of intuition. Then you will see that life has a meaning and that no matter what you are doing the inner voice is guiding you. That voice has long been drowned in the mire of untrue thoughts. The surest way to liberate the expression of intuition is by meditation, early in the morning and before going to bed at night.[98]

Advice and Resources

A wide range of established and more recent physical and psychological therapy methods is available. As we have explored in this book, none of these therapy methods can ever claim to help everybody at all times. This is also true for this book. The views expressed, and the practices suggested, come out of my personal and professional experience. As such they will be appropriate for some people some of the time. Unfortunately we are living in times, when many goods and services are being sold as the total solution. That can never be true.

So, if you want help with a psychological problem you will be best helped by someone who has experience with a wide range of such problems. If the material in this book has spoken to you, then you may also want to consider looking for someone with a spiritual perspective. The addresses below are all of bona fide organisations. In the U.K. you may want to check with your General Practitioner (Family Doctor). They often know the local 'scene' of counsellors and psychotherapists.

If you have any questions about the material in this book, or you would like to purchase Reinhard Kowalski's MindBalancing Relaxation & Meditation audio tape, please contact:

The Sattva Center
PO Box 2037, Maidenhead, Berks. SL6 3GZ, UK
www.sattvacenter.co.uk
E-mail: reinhard@sattvacenter.co.uk

1. Counsellors and Psychotherapists in the U.K.

If you are looking for a properly trained and accredited counsellor or psychotherapist in the U.K., contact these two professional bodies:

British Association for Counselling (BAC)
1 Regent Place, Rugby, Warks. CV21 2PJ
Telephone: +44 (0) 1788 550899 Fax: +44 (0) 1788 562189
E-mail :bac@bac.co.uk
www.bac.co.uk

United Kingdom Council for Psychotherapy (UKCP)
167-169 Great Portland Street, London W1N 5FB
Tel: +44 (0)20 7436 3002 Fax: +44 (0)20 7436 3013
E-mail: ukcp@psychotherapy.org.uk
www.psychotherapy.org.uk

If you would like to search for a psychosynthesis psychotherapist, contact:

The Institute of Psychosynthesis
65A Watford Way, Hendon, London NW4 3AQ
Telephone: +44 (0)20 8202 4525 Fax:+44 (0)20 8202 6166
E-Mail: institute@psychosynthesis.org

Psychosynthesis & Education Trust
92/94 Tooley Street, London SE1 2TH
Tel: +44 (0)20 7403 2100 Fax: +44 (0)20 7403 5562
E-mail: psychosynthesis.eductrust@btinternet.com

ReVision
97 Brondesbury Road, London NW6 6RY
Tel: +44 (0)20 8357 8881
E-mail: ReVision@cwcom.net

2. AYURVEDA RESOURCES

If you would like to find out more about training in, and literature about Ayurveda, here are three contacts.

For a two-year part-time training course in Ayurveda in the U.K. contact:

The College of Ayurveda (UK)
20 Annes Grove, Great Linford, Milton Keynes MK14 5DR
Tel.: +44 (0)1908 664518 Fax: +44 (0)870 0567947

In the U.S. Dr Vasant Lad runs a one-year intensive training course in Ayurveda. His Institute also offers books and Ayurvedic herbal remedies:

The Ayurvedic Institute
P.O. Box 23445, Albuquerque, N.M. 87192- 1445
Tel.: 505 291 9698 Fax: 505 294 7572
www.ayurveda.com

Dr David Frawley offers excellent correspondence courses in Ayurvedic Healing and in Vedic Astrology. His Institute is:

The American Institute of Vedic Studies
P.O. Box 8357, Santa Fe, N.M. 87504-8357
Tel.: 505 983 9385 Fax: 505 982 5807
www.vedanet.com

There is now also a European Academy of Ayurveda, offering treatment and training:

Mahindra Institute
Forsthausstrasse 6, 63633 Birstein, Germany
Tel.: +49 (0)6054 91310 Fax: +49 (0)6054 913136
www.ayurveda-academy.de

3. SPIRITUAL PATH AND YOGA

If you would like to find out more about the teaching of Paramahansa Yogananda, contact:

Self-Realization Fellowship
3880 San Rafael Avenue, Los Angeles, CA 90065 3298
Tel.: 323 225 2471 Fax: 323 225 5088
www.yogananda-srf.org

There are SRF meditation groups worldwide. If you contact the international headquarter in Los Angeles, they can put you in touch with a local group.

If you would like to explore Buddhist meditation practices in the U.K., contact:

Gaia House
West Ogwell, Newton Abbot, Devon TQ12 6EN
Tel.: +44 (0)1626 333613
www.gn.apc.org/gaiahouse/

Gaia House run excellent meditation courses at their centre and in other locations. Their website contains links to other Buddhist organisations worldwide.

Glossary of Sanskrit Terms

Ahamkara	The universal process of separation and differentiation. At an individual level it is the personal ego and the mental faculty and process of individuation, separation that creates the sense of 'I'.
Apana	The downward moving prana.
Astral	The astral body is our subtle body of impressions and prana. The astral plane is where souls go after death. Our most direct connection with the astral is through the chakras (subtle energy centres along the spine), and through the practice of yoga.
Ayurveda	'Science of life' – the yogic science of physical and mental healing.
Bhakti yoga	'Union through devotion' – the practice of devotional disciplines like worship, prayer, chanting in order to awaken love in the heart and connect with universal (God's) love.
Buddhi	Intelligence that is characterised by discrimination, calmness, contentment and forgiveness – the intelligence of the soul, which is the pole of the mind that is attracted towards sat (the real, truth, good).
Chakras	The energy centres of the subtle body are located along the spine and correspond to nerve plexuses and glands of the physical body. They are the gateway to the subtle body.
Gunas	The three prime qualities of nature – sattva, rajas and tamas.
Guru	Spiritual guide and teacher.
Karma	The law of cause and effect in Hinduism – means that all the actions of an individual will have corresponding effects stretching over several lifetimes.
Mahat	The divine mind or cosmic intelligence.
Manas	The outer mind or sense-mind.
Mantra	A 'mystic formula' – sound, syllable or word that has special powers and is used for yogic healing.

Maya	The cosmic creative force, the principle of manifestation, the principle of ever-changing matter. Also the illusory aspect of material reality, which blinds souls to the transcendent truth.
Prakriti	Primary matter, nature; one of the two supreme beginningless realities – the other one being purusha.
Prana	The vital force or vital air, moving in the human body as five primary life currents or vayus: prana, apana, vyana, udana and samana.
Pranayama	Control or expansion of the vital force through pranayama techniques.
Purusha	The transcendent Self. In the Sankhya system one of the two supreme beginningless realities, spirit or the male principle, whereas prakriti is the female principle or matter.
Rajas	One of the three gunas – the principle of action.
Sankhya	'Enumeration' – a philosophical system that is concerned with the tangible spectrum of creation. It identifies 25 elements including the gunas, prakriti and purusha.
Sattva	One of the three gunas – the principle of harmony and balance.
Tamas	One of the three gunas – the principle of darkness, stagnation and inertia.
Vedas	'Wisdom' – ancient sagely revelations about Self and cosmos, which are Hinduism's most authoritative scriptures.

Notes

1 Brian Swimme, *The Hidden Heart of the Cosmos,* Orbis Books, New York, 1996, p.110

2 Ibid., p.93

3 Satguru Sivaya Subramuniyaswami, *Dancing with Siva*, Himalayan Academy, India, USA, 1993, p.528

4 Paramahansa Yogananda, *Man's Eternal Quest*, Self-Realization Fellowship, Los Angeles, 1992, pp. 3-4

5 Douglas Grant Duff Ainslie in the preface to Paramahansa Yogananda, *The Science of Religion*, first published in 1953, p.X

6 Brother Achalananda in *A World in Transition*, Self-Realization Fellowship, Los Angeles, 1999, p.88

7 Brother Anandamoy in *A World in Transition*, pp. 39-40

8 Paramahansa Yogananda, *God talks with Arjuna – The Bhagavad Gita*, Self Realization Fellowship, 1995, Los Angeles.

9 Vasant Lad, *The Complete Book of Ayurvedic Home Remedies*, Harmony Books, New York, 1998, p.7

10 David Frawley, *Yoga and Ayurveda*, Lotus Press, Twin Lakes, 1999, pp. 20–21

11 Paramahansa Yogananda, *God talks with Arjuna – The Bhagavad Gita*, p.340

12 David Frawley, *Ayurvedic Healing Correspondence Course*, American Institute of Vedic Studies, Santa Fe, 1996, p.12

13 David Frawley, *Yoga & Ayurveda*, p.263

14 Christopher Thomson, *Nature and Human Nature*, Article on the website of The Medical and Scientific Network, 1989: http://www.cis.plym.ac.uk/SciMedNet/library/articles/9804202206.htm

15 Paramahansa Yogananda, *God talks with Arjuna – The Bhagavad Gita*, p.956

16 Emmanuel's Book II, *The Choice for Love*, Bantam Books, New York, 1989, pp. 3-4

17   The Independent on Sunday, 19.10.1997, quoting the Henley Centre's Media Futures Report.

18   Samuel H. Sandweiss, *Sai Baba – The Holy Man and the Psychiatrist*, Birth Day Publishing Company, San Diego, 1975, pp. 62-63

19   James Redfield, *The Celestine Prophecy*, Bantam Books, New York, 1994

20   Irvin Laszlo, *Life – A Dance through the Zero – Field*, in Caduceus, Issue 38, December 1997, p.16

21   Brian Swimme, *The Hidden Heart of the Cosmos*, p.96 – 103

22   Paramahansa Yogananda, *God talks with Arjuna – The Bhagavad Gita*, p.890

23   Vivekananda, *The Yogas and Other Works*, Ramakrishna- Vivekananda Center, New York, 1984, pp. 251-2

24   David Frawley, *Ayurveda and the Mind*, Lotus Press, Twin Lakes, 1996, p.54

25   Ken Wilber, *No Boundary*, Shambhala, Boston, 1979, pp. 17-18

26   Vasant Lad, *The Complete Book of Ayurvedic Home Remedies*, Harmony Books, New York, 1998, p.7

27   Vivekananda, *The Yogas and other Works*, Ramakrishna- Vivekananda Center, New York, 1984, p.471

28   Paramahansa Yogananda, *God talks with Arjuna – The Bhagavad Gita*, pp.145-46

29   M. Scott Peck, *The Road Less Traveled*, Arrow, New York, 1990

30   Paramahansa Yogananda, *God talks with Arjuna – The Bhagavad Gita*, p.184/85

31   Sri Daya Mata in *Self-Realization*, magazine published by Self- Realization Fellowship, Los Angeles, Spring 1998, p.24

32   Michael Talbot, *The Holographic Universe,* HarperPerennial, New York, 1992, p.79/80

33   Stanislav Grof, *The Cosmic Game,* Newleaf, Dublin, 1998

34   Stanislav Grof, *The Holotropic Mind*, Harper & Row, San Francisco, 1992, pp.29-30

35   Ibid., p.25

36   Ibid., p.77

37   Ken Wilber, *No Boundary*, Shambhala, Boston, 1979, pp.19-20

38   Ibid., p.21

39   Ibid., 1979, pp.48-49

40   Paramahansa Yogananda, *God talks with Arjuna -- The Bhagavad Gita*, p.957

41   Erich Fromm, *To Have or to Be*, Continuum, New York, 1997, p.1

42   Ibid, p.3

43   *The Independent on Sunday*, 11 October 1998, p.3

44   Paramahansa Yogananda, *The Science of Religion*, Self-Realization Fellowship, Los Angeles, 1982, pp.26-28

45   Erich Fromm (ed.), *Marx's Concept of Man*, Continuum, New York, 1992, p.3

46   Ibid., p.10

47   Ibid., p.10

48   Swami Akhilananda, *Hindu Psychology – Its Meaning for the West*, Routledge & Kegan Paul, London, 1960, p.216

49   Ben Elton, *Gridlock*, Sphere Books, London, 1992, p. 2,3,4

50   Rupert Sheldrake, The Rebirth of Nature, *Kindred Spirit*, 2(3), 16, 1991

51   Paramahansa Yogananda, *The Science of Religion*, p.29

52   Ken Wilber, *No Boundary*, Shambhala, Boston, 1979, pp.117-118

53   Ibid., 1979, pp.250-253

54   Roberto Assagioli, *Psychosynthesis*, Turnstone Press, Wellingborough, 1965, p.17- 24

55   Roberto Assagioli, *Transpersonal Development*, Crucible, London, 1991, pp.251-252

56   M. Lindfield, *The Dance of Change*, Arkana, London, 1986, p.165

57   Roberto Assagioli, *Transpersonal Development*, p.213

58   Ibid., pp.222-224

59   Stanislav Grof, *The Cosmic Game*, Newleaf, Dublin, 1998, p.114

60   Paramahansa Yogananda, *The Divine Romance*, Self-Realization Fellowship, Los Angeles, 1986, p.114

61   Paramahansa Yogananda, *Spiritual Diary*, Self Realization Fellowship, Los Angeles, 1989, entry for October 30

62   Paramahansa Yogananda, *The Law of Success*, Self- Realization Fellowship, Los Angeles, 1999, pp.23-4

63   David Frawley, *Ayurveda and the Mind*, Lotus Press, Twin Lakes, 1997, p.137

64   *The Upanishads*, Vedanta Press, Hollywood, 1983, p.37

65   This is the area that behavioural and cognitive therapy cover – see Reinhard Kowalski, *Discovering Your Self*, Routledge, London, 1993

66   Rob Weatherill, *Cultural Collapse*, Free Association Books, London, 1994 pp.77-78

67   Paramahansa Yogananda, *God talks with Arjuna – The Bhagavad Gita*, pp.184-5

68   Paramahansa Yogananda, *Man's Eternal Quest*, Self-Realization Fellowship, Los Angeles, 1992, p.175

69   Michael Talbot, *The Holographic Universe*, HarperPerennial, New York, 1992, p.138

70   David Frawley, *Ayurveda and the Mind*, Lotus Press, Twin Lakes, 1997, p.56

71   Paramahansa Yogananda, *The Divine Romance*, p.126

72   Mohan-Mala, *A Gandhian Rosary*, Navajivan Publishing House, Ahmedabad, 1993 p.59 (available from SRF, Los Angeles).

73   Swami Akhilananda, *Hindu Psychology – Its Meaning for the West*, Routledge & Kegan Paul, London, 1960, p.76

74   Arthur C. Clarke and Michael Kube-McDowell put forward a fascinating hypothesis in their recent novel *The Trigger*, HarperCollins, London, 1999, p.414: 'In this new and provocative view, the Big Bang was not the birth of the Universe, but the birth of its consciousness.' This corresponds with my considerations.

75   Vasant Lad, Mano Vaha Srotas, *Ayurveda Today*, The Ayurvedic Institute, Albuquerque,Vol.XI, No.2, 1999, p.5

76   Paramahansa Yogananda, *Autobiography of a Yogi*, Self-Realization Fellowship, Los Angeles, 1981, pp.238-40. Kriya Yoga is the core technique taught by Yogananda in his lessons, which can be obtained from SRF. The technique is very powerful and requires the teaching and guidance that is available in the SRF lessons. The breathing techniques in this book and in the MindBalancing practice are not Kriya Yoga as taught by SRF.

77   More about breathing exercises and counting can be found in: William Bloom, *Meditation in a Changing World*, Gothic Image Publications, Glastonbury, 1987; Satguru Sivaya Subramuniyaswami, *Merging with Siva*, Himalayan Academy, Hawaii, 1999, p.168; David Frawley, *Yoga and Ayurveda*, Lotus Press, Twin Lakes, 1999, pp.251ff.

78   David Frawley, *Ayurvedic Healing*, Passage Press, Salt Lake City, 1989, p.xix

79   Satguru Sivaya Subramuniyaswami, *Dancing with Siva*, Himalayan Academy, India, USA, 1993, p.693

80   Mike King, 'God, Science and Jnani: a New Framework', *Network* 71, The Scientific and Medical Network, 1999

81   David Frawley, *Ayurveda and the Mind*, Lotus Press, Twin Lakes, 1997, p.245

82   Sri Daya Mata, *Enter the Quiet Heart*, Self-Realization Fellowship, Los Angeles, 1998, pp.43-46

83   See, for example, *Anxiety and Stress Management Toolkit*, Winslow, Bicester, 1999; *Relaxation Tools CD*, Joliko, Maidenhead 1997. Contact the Sattva Center for further details.

84   Paramahansa Yogananda, *Where There Is Light*, Self-Realization Fellowship, Los Angeles, p.86

85   David Frawley, *Ayurveda and the Mind*, Lotus Press, Twin Lakes, 1997, p.115

86   Ibid., p.151

87   Reinhard Kowalski, *Anxiety and Stress Management Toolkit*, Winslow, Bicester, 1999

88   This is the definition of the gunas as found in the famous translation by Sir Edwin Arnold, *The Song Celestial or Bhagavad Gita*, Self-Realization Fellowship, Los Angeles, 1989, p.153

89   David Frawley, *Ayurveda and the Mind*, p. 34/35

90   David Frawley, *Yoga and Ayurveda*, Lotus Press, Twin Lakes, 1999, p.32

91   Reprinted with permission from *Yoga and Ayurveda* by Dr. David Frawley, Lotus Press, P. O. Box 325,Twin Lakes, WI 53181. ©1999 All Rights Reserved.

92   David Frawley, *Ayurveda and the Mind*, p.229

93   Ibid., p.226

94   Paramahansa Yogananda, 'The God-given Purpose and Potentials of the Human Body- Temple', *Self Realization Magazine*, Self-Realization Fellowship, Los Angeles, Spring 2000, p.21

95   See David Frawley, *Yoga and Ayurveda*, pp.251ff for more details

96   Paramahansa Yogananda in *Self Realization Magazine*, Spring 2000, p.20

97   Paramahansa Yogananda, *God talks with Arjuna – The Bhagavad Gita*, Self Realization Fellowship, Los Angeles, p. 311

98   Paramahansa Yogananda, *Journey to Self-Realization*, Self-Realization Fellowship, Los Angeles, 1997, pp.111-12

Index

The MindBalancing Meditation Programme
Courses and audio-cassette

In meditation you shut out the external world that you normally perceive with the senses. You also withdraw your attention from the constant stream of thoughts in your mind. You move from Manas, the outer mind of the senses, to Buddhi, the inner mind of the soul. According to Yoga and Ayurveda real healing of ourselves and of our world can only happen from the inner mind of the soul, which is our true Self.

We are living in a world that is dominated by hectic activity, increasing speed, greed and attachments to external objects and goals. Yoga states that this focus on seeking pleasure in the outer world brings with it its flip side, which is misery, lethargy, fear, depression. The only way out of the up and down of what we call 'modern living' is to re-connect with that deep place of stillness inside, which is our soul. Meditation is the key to it.

Meditation is best learned in a group setting because of the support and energy that are created when people learn and meditate together. The Sattva Center is running four-week courses consisting of five one-and-a-half hour group sessions. The courses teach the MindBalancing meditation and relaxation programme which has grown from this book and is described in Chapter 11.

Reinhard Kowalski has also recorded an audio-cassette with the MindBalancing relaxation and meditation exercises. The cassette comes with a detailed introduction to yoga meditation on the inlay card. It is used as the practice tape on the Sattva Center courses.

Please contact the Sattva Center if you are interested in attending one of our courses, or would like us to run a meditation course in your work or social setting. You can also purchase the MindBalancing tape from us for your individual practice.

> The Sattva Center
> PO Box 2037
> Maidenhead, Berks. SL6 3GZ, U.K.
> e-mail: courses@sattvacenter.co.uk

In the United States you can purchase the MindBalancing audio-cassette from:
> Wellness Reproductions & Publishing Inc.
> 23945 Mercantile Road
> Beachwood, Ohio 44122-5924
> http://www.wellness-resources.com

Understanding Reality

A Commonsense Theory of the Original Cause

Stefan Hlatky and Philip Booth

A bold attempt to break through the limitations of traditional philosophy and theology, by learning from our everyday experience and commonsense.

Hlatky's thesis is that we cannot understand our own lives unless we understand the reality that we live in, and we cannot understand the reality we live in unless we understand its original cause.

By contrast, the original cause has traditionally been treated as two questions: *what is the origin of our own existence on Earth?* and *what is the origin of the Earth and the universe?* Hlatky argues his hypothesis that the original cause is a non-created living being, a whole, of which we are non-created parts.

He follows tradition in calling that whole 'God', but argues, unusually, that God has the same need that we and every living being have: to be understood, and thereby to be loved. This need motivates God to give out creation: he wants to be understood by us. Through connecting with a body provided for us by God in creation, we can come to an understanding of our relationship to God and to each other, with huge consequences for the way we live our lives.

Hlatky argues his view on the basis of our experience of everyday reality, in other words on the basis of the self-evident, the commonsense. On this basis, he criticises the illogicalities in traditional theological and pantheist or New Age views, as well as in the stance of modern science. He lays out the implications of his hypothesis for many pressing human problems: love and the nature of relationships, education and child-rearing, morals and ethics, political organization, the environment, the role and limits of science, etc.

This book, which contains original articles by Hlatky and dialogues between the two authors, cuts across conventional disciplines and will be of interest to anyone who is curious about the big questions of life.

Stefan Hlatky is a retired lawyer, born in Hungary and now living in Sweden. **Philip Booth** is a psychotherapist living in Oxford.

£13 paperback   256pp   1 897766 42 4

Sex, Spirit and Community

Mark Josephs-Serra

The relationship between our inner journeys and our politics is of profound, crucial importance. Bizarre or radical as it may seem at first, this book looks at how a more sacred sexuality, a more engaged spirituality, and a greater honouring of ourselves and others can become the foundations of deep community.

There was spirituality and unity in traditional culture, but also rigidity and repression. Modern culture is characterised by sexual freedom and individuality, but also by emptiness and fragmentation. Sex, Spirit and Community is a passionate and intelligent book from the cutting edge of the holistic cultural trend to be found throughout contemporary society – in green awareness, in health foods, in self-development and alternative economic strategies.

Moving towards a vision of a more decentralised society, the author addresses the question of how to develop communities that acknowledge the mystery of life and death, the magnificence of the earth, and the importance of love, hate, joy and fear – not only in our inner worlds, but in the way we organise our practical, everyday lives.

Mark Josephs-Serra looks at repression of the body, repression of the spirit, and repression of the heart. His book is about a journey towards personal wholeness, towards community structures that can bond us in a sense of a shared journey, and towards political organisation rooted in a commitment to that shared journey.

Mark Josephs-Serra was born a Jew, but after a decade as a Hindu monk he has spent many years reconnecting with the earth and studying the art of relationships. His organisation 'Balance' has involved hundreds of people in exploring deep, holistic community.

£9.95 paperback   224pp   1 897766 60 2

Life Style

A Parable of Sharing

A. H. Dammers

Horace Dammers explores the structural connection between our personal and individual use of the earth's resources, and the great issues of peace, justice and the environment. He poses Kant's three fundamental questions, What Can I Know?, What Ought I to Do?, and What May I Hope? in the context of a rich examination of the biblical tradition and the relevance of its teachings for today. A simple lifestyle would, he believes, release both the resources and energies necessary for social change: Jesus' poverty was not an affliction but a strength, and as such forms the core of his teachings about lifestyle.

The author states the need for simplicity of lifestyle in the face of the demands of a global capitalist consumerist culture. He shows how the foundation and growth of the Life Style Movement — and other 'downshifting' movements of a similar kind — has provided the necessary mutual support for people determined in the face of all the odds to leave the world a better place than they find it.

After war service, **A. H. Dammers** was ordained a priest in the Church of England, serving in both Britain and India and becoming Dean of Bristol. In 1972 he founded the Life Style Movement which flourishes to this day. The first edition of *Life Style: A Parable of Sharing* was published in 1982.

"This book points a way to a simpler lifestyle in which the spiritual, psychological and aesthetic gains outweigh the loss of material luxuries... I hope nobody will read this book without taking a radical step or three."
Walter Schwarz in the Foreword

£11.99 paperback 192pp   1 897766 64 5

Good God

Green theology and the value of creation

Jonathan Clatworthy

Good God examines our inherited value judgements about the world, and their roots in different theories of creation. It explores the relationship between value judgements, cosmology and ethics, creating a theological justification for defending the natural order against ecological destruction. This 'green' agenda for social objectives is distinct from the left-right spectrum of modern political discourse.

By mercilessly exposing inconsistencies in the Christian tradition, the author undermines virtually the whole of what Christianity stands for in the modern West. In asking what it is about modern technological society that makes us so determined to destroy our natural environment, he puts the blame largely on the mechanistic paradigm of modern secular thought. Paradoxically, he then uses modern biblical scholarship to show how this alternative account, often condemned as pagan, is in fact a major theme of the Bible. By analysing both the world-affirming and the world-denying elements of the Christian tradition, he develops a 'Green theology' — a distinctive account of how we and the world relate to God that sheds light on the issues of environmental debate and constitutes a major challenge to Western society to make radical changes to its values.

Jonathan Clatworthy is an anglican priest with parish experience in Manchester, Sheffield and Staffordshire. He is a council member of the Modern Churchpeople's Union, and in 1991 founded the journal *Theology in Green* (now published as Ecotheology by Sheffield Academic Press).

'A bold and wide-ranging essay, reinforcing the need to be clearer about our basic valuation of the world. Pessimism or would-be 'neutrality' about the world offer no hope for transforming action, and the continuing crisis of the ecosystem should long since have woken us up to the urgency of re-examining how we value our environment.' Rowan Williams, Bishop of Monmouth

'Lucid, well-argued and exciting.' Walter Schwarz, author and journalist

'Proposes an optimistic valuing of the world as God's creation, and that in turn leads to actions of co-operation rather than competition. A coherent theological basis for green ethics.' Dr Ruth Page, Dept of Theology and Religious Studies, University of Edinburgh

£13 pbk   240pp   1 897766 37 8

ALSO PUBLISHED BY JON CARPENTER

Our books may be ordered from bookshops or (post free) from
Jon Carpenter Publishing, Alder House, Market Street, Charlbury,
England OX7 3PH

For details of distributors in other parts of the world, please
e-mail carpenter@oxfree.com

Credit card orders should be phoned or faxed to 01689 870437
or 01608 811969